PRAISE FOR *THE LANGUAGE YOUR BODY SPEAKS*

"As physicians trained to only practice and value the objectivity of evidence-based medicine, we tend to dismiss the subjective aspects of healing — things like intuition, the emotional realm, the flow of life force through our bodies, and the stories we tell ourselves — which can make us sick or help cure disease. In medical school nobody taught me to pay attention to the unique language of my body or the bodies of my patients, to tune in to how sound, color, touch, my environment, my connection to the spiritual realms, or my thoughts, beliefs, and feelings might affect physical health. Lucky for us, Ellen Meredith picks up where evidence-based medicine leaves off, guiding us into the subjective aspects of healing with an obviously masterful synthesis of many healing methods that should be included in medical education but aren't. For the scientists and skeptics, this book will be a stretch because this material is unapologetically unprovable. But for those willing to stay open to and curious about the art and mystery of healing, especially those whom evidence-based medicine has failed to help, this book is just what the doctor ordered."

— **Lissa Rankin, MD,** *New York Times* bestselling author of *Mind Over Medicine* and founder of the Whole Health Medicine Institute

"This book is destined to be on the top of your reference stack. Again and again you'll reach for it when you're curious about what your body is telling you or when you want more insight. The wisdom here is incredible and the exercises are just right for discovering your own personal language that your body is speaking. Ellen Meredith gives you the very tools you need to unlock this language that is waiting patiently for your arrival for your own personal miracles."

— **Lauren Walker,** creator and author of *The Energy Medicine Yoga Prescription*

"*The Language Your Body Speaks* is a treasure! Ellen Meredith's clear description of how to recognize, decode, and heal the body's subtle energy systems is an accessible pathway to maximum vitality for everyone, regardless of age or background. Having atter⸺⸺⸺⸺ ⸺f Ellen's workshops, I know the amazing value these tec⸺ and for my students and clients."

— **Devi Stern, MS, EEM-AP,** author of *Ener⸺*

"Brilliant! Ellen Meredith guides the reader through *The Language Your Body Speaks* on an experiential journey of self-discovery and healing. Ellen weaves an energetic tapestry that awakens you into a deeper experience of the soul. It's powerful both for beginners and for energy medicine practitioners, who can learn to listen to their innate wisdom and dialogue using the 'language the body speaks.'"

— **Dr. Melanie Smith**, DOM, AP, EEM-AP of
Well Within Natural Medicine, Inc., and author of
the Energy Mastery for Healthy Living online series

"This warm, rich, informative, and generous book is essential reading both for practitioners and for those who would like to unlock the healing power of energy in their lives."

— **Dawson Church**, bestselling author of *The Genie in Your Genes*

"This book will coach you to look at illness and wellness in a new way so your life can be a journey full of health and joy!"

— **Dondi Dahlin**, bestselling author of *The Five Elements*
and coauthor of *The Little Book of Energy Medicine*

"Ellen Meredith never disappoints, and this book is an absolute must-have for anyone who takes their energy medicine seriously, who wants to learn the language of their body's energies to truly empower their self-care. Drawing from ancient wisdom and her own experience, she effortlessly weaves and creates protocols that get results and that are enjoyable to do, which means you will do them! Don't hesitate to make this part of your library — you won't regret it."

— **Madison King**, writer and teacher

"Since awareness is curative, knowing what the body is saying spontaneously triggers the healing process. In a world bursting with information, *The Language Your Body Speaks* is a drop of pure wisdom."

— **Jacob Liberman**, OD, PhD, author of *Luminous Life*

The Language
Your Body Speaks

The Language
Your Body Speaks

Self-Healing
with Energy Medicine

ELLEN MEREDITH

Foreword by Donna Eden

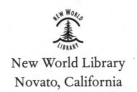

New World Library
Novato, California

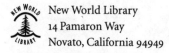 New World Library
14 Pamaron Way
Novato, California 94949

Figures 3, 4, 8, 18, 19, and 20 by Tracy Cunningham

Text design by Tona Pearce Myers

Library of Congress Cataloging-in-Publication data is available.

First printing, May 2020
ISBN 978-1-60868-675-9
Ebook ISBN 978-1-60868-676-6
Printed in Canada on 100% postconsumer-waste recycled paper

 New World Library is proud to be a Gold Certified Environmentally Responsible Publisher. Publisher certification awarded by Green Press Initiative.

10   9   8   7   6   5   4   3   2

To all you self-healers who are willing to think outside the box and enter into energy dialogue with your own being.

You don't have to be sick to learn how to cultivate well-being. But if you are chronically ill, I believe the best path to healing is to learn how to encode wellness in each moment of your life. May the material in this book help to awaken your own understandings and ability to communicate with all dimensions of yourself.

CONTENTS

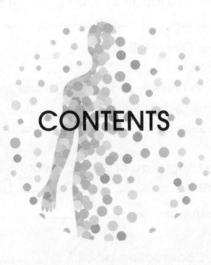

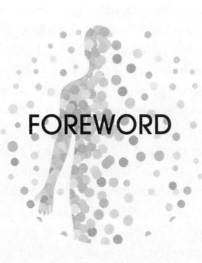

FOREWORD

Imagine what your life would feel like if you could access the archives of knowledge that lie within the energies of your body. It would awaken something wonderful inside, an empowerment and sense of wonder and awe about life…along with gratitude and pure joy about the miracle of it all. Life would be better.

I love Ellen Meredith's book, *The Language Your Body Speaks*. It is a great guide to understanding what we once knew organically as babies. Before we learned the language of words, we knew the language of energy. As babies, we were attuned to our own energies and the energies of our caregivers. This book can teach you how to know the language of energy again and even speak it!

Energy flows everywhere in and out of our bodies; it is the foundation for everything physical. It orchestrates everything in our lives, from emotions to digestion to getting ourselves out of bed in the morning and going to bed at night.

Without energy, our bodies would be like cars with no fuel. Without energy, we aren't alive.

Ellen believes we are all storytellers, and she encourages rich dialogue with the stories we carry inside, which can inform and heal us. Physical ailments cannot be separated from your emotions and mental processes. We are body, mind, spirit, and soul. By deciphering the language of energy and uncovering deep meaning and answers to why your body is hurting or your mind is tormented, you will not only be freed from pain, but you will also learn the language to delve into your body's mysteries forevermore.

This lovely book will teach you how to use everything inside you, from your mind and intuition to your senses and elements, and finally to moving your hands to connect with and shift your own energies.

I met Ellen Meredith in 2007 in a class I was teaching on energy medicine. She was already an energy healer of many years, but as a great teacher with an open mind, she embraced being a beginner again, allowing the training to expand her experience of life and teaching.

Like most of us in energy medicine, Ellen's fascination with energy never ends. So connecting up with others on the same wavelength was a fruitful continuation of her journey to understand energy.

I have read a lot of books on energy over the years — but Ellen's is different. It is a breath of fresh air, and I believe it is necessary. Ellen respects and supports each person's own inner guidance to finding solutions, and so this is not merely a book of techniques. Ellen clearly and beautifully shares how to talk energy and figure out what to do to heal.

She liberates students from identifying too much with their own suffering. She instead encourages curiosity about our wondrous bodies and fun in discovering what a physical ailment might mean. Because she understands that we are each unique beings and can be very creative in the poignancy and drama of our own wounds, she teaches the reader how to be a storyteller of their wounds to themselves. She offers techniques that help us enter into our own psyches and energies for healing. As Ellen says, "The goal of this work is not to fix your energies but to encounter them and have a heartfelt, loving, supportive dialogue." *The Language Your Body Speaks* teaches you to trust your body and know it as your partner.

Weaving insights from ancient cultures, her teachers, and her own council, Ellen invites you to commune with the vast intelligence at work inside you and become emotionally congruent and deeply satisfied.

I stand in awe of Ellen's gift for putting ideas into words.

She is a visionary who is committed to sharing her wisdom with everyone. This book opens, expands, and enhances a person's existence into a much better lifetime than they were having. It is masterful.

I think one of the best things about this book is the realization that consciousness is a whole-body phenomenon. When something goes wrong with your body, it is a welcome relief to know you can converse with it and find out why your body did this, what it might mean, and what you can do to heal yourself. It is empowering. It is freeing. And it can change your life forever.

Enjoy,
Donna Eden,
author of *Energy Medicine*

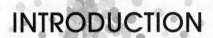

INTRODUCTION

The Language Your Body Speaks

Energy is the language your body speaks.

— Donna Eden

True confession: I am a language geek. When I was twelve, I used to sit for hours listening to foreign radio programs. The rhythms and cadences and sounds would thrill me. The sense that there was a conversation I could *almost* understand pulled me in. The music of it spoke to me. It filled and satisfied me in ways that the programs in English, talking about boring everyday things, did not.

My mother thought I was crazy. She'd say, "Why are you wasting your time with that? You don't know what they are saying." I'd say, "But on some level I do know. I *can* understand them." She would shake her head and go back to her housework. And I would dive back into the thrill of the barely understood rivers of sound.

Some years later I studied many of those languages and found I still had that liminal sense of understanding, even when I didn't know for sure, with my logical brain, what the words all meant. Learning foreign languages felt like I was remembering something I'd known in another life. I wondered if there was some kind of source code underlying the specifics of each tongue that I could understand even if I didn't know the vocabulary or grammar rules.

It is no wonder that fifty-plus years later I have written a book titled *The Language Your Body Speaks*. This book is about using the language of energy to take care of yourself, to participate in the conversations between your body, spirit, and mind, and to heal yourself. In the many years since my foreign radio adventures, I've had opportunities to track down some of that source code I was feeling, our first language of energy expressing itself, and become more fluent. I've spent the last thirty-five years working as a professional energy medicine practitioner and intuitive, helping clients learn to participate more fruitfully in their own body, mind, and spirit conversations.

ENERGY AS A LANGUAGE

Most of us talk about energy in practical terms. We say, "She's got great energy," meaning we sense from subtle cues that someone is animated or perhaps particularly comfortable to be around. We say, "I don't have the energy to argue right now," meaning that activity is somehow not being funded, emotionally, physically, or even spiritually. We say, "My energy has crashed," meaning we have run out of fuel. On an intuitive level, learning about the subtle energies that we are composed of and how to positively influence their behaviors makes a lot of sense.

Your body is made up of energies. What appears to be solidly physical — the cells, the bones, the tissue, the organs — is in fact a swirling, moving set of energetic exchanges. Even the chemical processes of your body are energetic at their root: Chemistry is the story of energetic exchanges at the molecular level.

And just under the surface of your awareness, your body, mind, and spirit are using a language of energetic signaling to communicate constantly with one another.

Using a vocabulary of light, sound, vibration, imagery, sensation, and other messaging, your body, mind, and spirit are talking with one another, adjusting your physical self to match your thoughts, influencing your thoughts to recognize the needs of your body, and embodying the urgings of your spirit. There is a grammar to this language: patterns of movement and energetic exchange. Like all languages, the subtle energies that you are made of encode meaning and shape your experience.

Is learning the language of energy really necessary? It is crucial if you want to be able to participate in your own evolving experience and create the life you crave. Imbalance in the body, mind, or spirit communicates through symptoms, feelings, sensations, thoughts, and events. If we miss those communiqués, the body and mind shout louder and discomfort snowballs into illness.

I learned this truth the hard way. My path to becoming a healer included a years-long slide into chronic illness that finally forced me to wake up and listen to what my body, mind, and spirit were trying to teach me.

Chronic health problems showed up early in my life. At first, they took the form of minor ailments, frequent ankle sprains, and stomach upsets. Then my weight ballooned when I skipped third grade and turned to sugar for consolation, after losing my friends. That led to blood sugars careening wildly, leaving me alternately too animated or too crashed out.

Where did all this tumult come from? In part, I was a sensitive kid living in a family rife with unnamed, unacknowledged conflict. My parents were camouflaging difficulties in a marriage that didn't work. They were just too different. My mother's core value was "never do anything in excess." If I got hurt, her response was, "Oh, I'm sure you are fine." My father, on the other hand, was grandiose and brilliant, though emotionally clueless. His response to my complaints was to brag that he had never had a day of illness in his life. Clearly, he believed that anything true for him should be true for his offspring. Conflicts in style, worldview, and values are common in families. These often give rise to the internal, sometimes invisible existential stress of a soul that feels unrecognized, setting the stage for chronic illness. If Mom was a violin, Dad was a tuba. So how was I to learn to take care of my oboe self and really play my instrument?

As my mom was trying to get me to rosin my bow and tune my nonexistent strings, my father was saying, "We're both wind instruments, so just go *oom-pah, oom-pah,* and you'll get along great." And there I was, an oboe, filling the tube with phlegm and not knowing enough to shake it out. I was desperately trying to play the music of my soul on an instrument I never learned how to manage properly.

I careened through my early years with weight fluctuations, food obsessions, mild flu-like symptoms, and allergies, and I spent hours under the covers reading and ruining my eyesight. This led to hormone imbalances in adolescence, depression, and chronic dieting and bingeing. And my poor soggy oboe degenerated with bouts of compulsive exercise, rounds of fatigue that might last for months, and behavior that ranged between overanimation and depression. By the time I was nearing thirty, the situation had degenerated into daily migraines and a vulnerability to viruses, parasites, and other beasties that would disrupt my energies' ability to communicate and function for months at a time. Not a pretty picture!

None of the many physicians I consulted ever found anything medically wrong with me. In fact, most of them implied that it was normal for hormones and moods to swing, or they labeled my issues a function of personality and therefore an emotional problem.

Then finally I ran into a doctor who woke me up with a simple truth. I went to see her with severe digestive discomfort and ongoing exhaustion. She conducted numerous tests, examined me thoroughly, and gave me a diagnosis of blinding clarity: I had "malaise."

I was furious. *Malaise* is French for "discomfort." She charged me eighty dollars to tell me I had discomfort! But like all truths, it wormed its way past my anger to stick in my brain. She said, "Medicine" — meaning allopathic, Western medicine — "has nothing to offer you. I'm going to give you the name and number of a complementary medicine practitioner who might be able to help."

In retrospect, malaise was exactly what I had. I had no idea how to bring comfort, specific to my particular mind-body, moment by moment, hour by hour, day by day. And my body was registering its objections with louder and louder cries for help.

During all those years of pain and dysfunction, I wish I'd known that the body speaks its truth through symptoms — through sensations, through interruptions of functioning, through energetic blockages, through physical signals that say, *Pay attention, I need something here.* Those needs might be nourishment, safety, a different pace, compassion, help clearing or tuning the instrument, rest, release, connection, a different environment. And if we don't get the communication, the body shouts louder.

The communication may start small: a dip in energy that keeps us home from a party, or a somewhat sore throat, or an allergic reaction, or an achy joint, or loss of focus, or a slight miscommunication, mishap, or moment of misbehavior. Yet these messages *progress* if we don't really listen and respond. The symptoms get louder and more severe; processes and functioning are disrupted. Digestion, circulation, tissue repair, and/ or hormonal communication can falter. And the instrument progresses from malaise to malady (sickness), which also snowballs — sometimes because of the pharmaceuticals we take in lieu of authentic communication; sometimes because the habit of not knowing how to care for our own particular, beautiful, amazing instrument just wears it down over time.

A PATH TO HEALING

Although illness can be extremely complex, a compounding of years of miscommunication, the path to healing can be much simpler and more direct. If you learn the language of energy, learn to let your body, mind, and spirit communicate to you in their wisdom about what your instrument needs, and then provide that moment by moment, you will heal.

In the past thirty-five years, I've worked with thousands of clients, some with extremely complex and serious life-threatening medical conditions, and others with less dramatic, life-interrupting chronic symptoms. All of them were seeking ways to find support for their instrument rather than mere management of their symptoms or disease. I have seen, again and again, how powerfully you can activate healing once you participate in the ongoing communications of your body, mind, and spirit.

My path into healing work evolved from necessity. It was also shaped by some outside-the-box experiences that were not in the violin-tuba culture on offer in my home when I was growing up.

In my early twenties, my world cracked open. My beloved, but dead, grandmother, a woman who had been massively obese in her life, showed up in my mind's eye. She told me not to follow the path she had followed but instead to open to guidance. I was not sure what that meant. But within a day, I was seeing a ticker tape of letters scrolling through my head with a message from my inner teachers, group consciousnesses who called themselves my Councils.

Within a week, I was hearing that guidance in my mind, taking dictation on a rich curriculum of spiritual, perceptual energy training that continues to this day, forty-plus years later. You'd think that with all their wisdom, they could have kept me from getting sick! Instead, they predicted that I'd move to California, grow even sicker, and in the process of healing, become an energy healer.

They said, "We're going to give you three initial tools." I took dictation: "A golden sheaf of wheat, freshly cut. A solid earth stone. A pair of silver scissors." It made me giggle. I had no idea what they were for, and they sounded like props in a fairy tale.

Later that same day, however, there was a knock on my door. It was an acquaintance from school, a woman I barely knew, who said, "Are you a healer? I need some help."

Telling the story now, I'm not sure why I said, "Yes, come on in." I had only three tools and no clue what to do with them. But at the time, it seemed natural.

She explained what was going on. Her digestion was off, and she was having shooting pains in her arms and legs. She was in enough discomfort that she couldn't concentrate to do her schoolwork. She'd been to the doctor, who ran tests and told her nothing was wrong.

My memory of the actual session is a bit vague. I remember using the wheat to stir the air around her intestines and then to repeatedly pull energies out and shake them off. I remember placing the stone on her solar plexus, and she reported that it made her gut feel calm for the first time in months. I used the scissors to cut some lines that I then hooked up to other lines at the suggestion of my Councils. And I remember being on the brink of giggling the whole time. But step by step, my hands just proceeded, and in about thirty minutes, it was done.

She said, "Thank you, that did the trick. I feel much better." We never discussed it, although she did mention about a month later that the symptoms had never returned.

Looking back, I wonder why the whole experience didn't leave me shaken or confused. Maybe it was like my experiences of listening to foreign languages. I had the sense that I could *almost* understand it. And I was willing to listen and learn.

About eight months later, I did end up moving to California, as my Councils had predicted. I soaked up the sunshine and the go-with-the-flow culture and thrived for a few months, until I had another energy and nutritional crash, this time so serious I found it difficult to do simple tasks. This led me to the momentous diagnosis of malaise.

The complementary practitioner my doctor (bless her heart) referred me to was a chiropractor, who had studied a newly developed form of healing called Applied Kinesiology.

This chiropractor diagnosed me with a complex of things that have since become almost clichés in the complementary medicine world: candida imbalance in my gut, leaky gut, blood sugar imbalance, adrenal crash, and for the headaches that were starting to show up more frequently, cranial jamming. I was delighted to have names and explanations. But more, I was enchanted with the technique she called *muscle testing*, a biofeedback tool that allowed her to ask my body what was going on in various energy channels and get responses in the form of muscles holding strong or releasing.

Dialoguing with the body in this way made sense to me. I loved the Chinese medicine charts on her walls and the way she'd use these pathways to figure out what needed to be balanced in my body's energies. I had always thought of energy as what I didn't have when I crashed out. I had never thought of it as the fuel that governs the body's functions in positive ways!

Then something strange started happening to me. First, I found I could predict which meridian pathway would test "weak" with the muscle tests. I could just feel it, see it, or even hear it. My chiropractor used a lot of nutritional supplements and dietary modifications as part of her healing work. I discovered I could see which supplements I'd need. I could point to the bottle on the shelf that contained what I needed, and I could even tell her the ideal dosage. Although I knew so little about anatomy that I didn't even know where my organs were located, I found I could point to the organs that were out of balance, and the energy testing would confirm it. I could *see* in my mind's eye that my chiropractor's gallbladder was a lovely forest green and mine was puke green, and sure enough, my gallbladder meridian would test weak.

Over the course of the six months we worked together on my health, I learned to feel when an energy would test weak, and I started seeing what might fix it. Some of the fixes were in line with Applied Kinesiology. Others were more off the wall. For example, I might take both hands and push the energy on either side of my head down my body and off into the ground. Then an energy that had tested weak would right itself.

With time, my energies balanced, my gut healed, and my lifelong exploration of energy healing was launched.

SELF-HEALING WITH ENERGY MEDICINE

Energy medicine is, as Donna Eden and David Feinstein have said, a form of healing in which energy is both the patient *and* the medicine.[1] Our bodies communicate using chemical messaging and energetic messaging. By using energy techniques to influence the energetic messaging of the body, mind, and spirit, we can influence the behaviors of the body (including its chemistry) and activate its natural abilities to heal.

In its contemporary form, energy medicine involves using pathways and techniques mapped out within various traditions, such as Chinese medicine, Ayurvedic medicine, yoga, and shamanic healing, among others, in healing practices that date back thousands of years. Contemporary energy medicine also incorporates newer understandings from energy healing pioneers, physics, kinesiology, and body-mind modalities, which give us ways to work practically with our subtle energies to promote well-being.

In this book, I invite you to delve beneath the particulars of formal energy medicine modalities to understand the source codes, the language that underlies them. Too often people with chronic illness are drawn to study complementary modalities or nutritional science in a desperate search for wellness, but they end up learning dietary dictums and prescribed practices, rather than how to actually participate in the communications of their body, mind, and spirit. My goal in presenting this language is for you to be able to create your own, personalized energy medicine, in order to truly participate in your own creation of self. My goal in focusing on self-healing is to encourage you to discover how to take healing into your own hands and, in a very individualized way, support your miraculous, inbuilt capacity to heal.

ENERGY DIALOGUE

Energy dialogue is at the heart of successful energy medicine. It quite simply involves being able to get the messages from your body, spirit, and mind and to respond in their idiom — using movement, gesture, light, sound, vibration, imagery, interaction with energy flows, actions, placement in an environment, and more. This is the vocabulary of the language of energy.

The goal of energy dialogue is to participate moment by moment in the ongoing energy communications within you. It is not something to use just when you are sick. It is a practice that allows you to bring your body's rhythms and expressions, your conscious understanding, and your behaviors into collaboration, creating your spirit's truest embodiment.

Once you can participate in energy dialogue, you have the basis for activating and supporting your body's natural ability to heal.

You use energy dialogue much as you use any language. As you proceed through your day, consider all the ways you use language to think or speak. First, there are the monologues and imagined conversations going on in your head. Perhaps you listen to the radio as you get ready for work. You might have conversations with family members or talk to yourself in the mirror. You might interact with the neighbor on your way out the door, and so on. All of this is natural. You probably don't have to stop and formulate sentences, look up words in a dictionary, do fifteen minutes of language exercises, or struggle to find the right tone of voice or emphasis as you joke, question, respond, or inform.

The goal in learning the language of energy is to participate in the energetic dialogues that are *you* and to skillfully navigate among the exchanges with energies that are not you. If you are fluent in the language of energy, it becomes second nature to rebalance your energies, to pull in what is needed, and to recognize when something requires conscious attention.

USING ENERGY DIALOGUE THROUGHOUT THE DAY

The energies that make up your body continuously move and swirl and spiral and flow and block and release and swarm and envelop. They put on quite a show. If you have eyes to see, there are patterns to the movement and colors that represent differing vibrations or kinds of movement. There are shapes created by energies moving in collaborative ways. Some healers refer to this massive dance of energies as the *energy body*, and it has been mapped in various cultures. What is amazing is that, although you can find common features from one body to the next, each energy dance is also individual and unique.

And if you have ears to hear, it's a counterpoint of sounds, a symphony of exchanges embodying meaning, intention, and recognition. It is choruses engaged in call and response, expressing our truth. And each of us is set to a different, individualized key. There are harmonies and dissonance, melody lines and chords, and elements (like the heart) that set and keep the beat. It is extremely entertaining to tune in and just listen!

Imagine if, as a child, you learned to tune in to this dimension of being. Today, you would see, hear, feel, know, and smell when the patterns shifted or faltered. It would be no big deal to recognize what is needed and supply it, to recognize what is going awry and right it, to participate in that conversation as it is unfolding.

If you had learned this language as a child, your day might look something like this: You would wake up and spend a few minutes just checking in — helping the energies transition from the more muted circulation during sleep to the more active movement of your day. You would know if it's time to get up or you need more rest. You would feel what pace and rhythm is needed. You might stretch every which way to allow energies space to flow. You would hook up the main energy arteries that run up the front and back of the spine — like getting Main Street cleared of snow. You might tap or drum various junction points in your energy circulation system to get that system circulating more effectively.

As you get out of bed, you would check in to see if you are truly oriented to the energies around you — including those of the earth and sky. You would make sure that your elements are balanced. You might tune in to your spirit, your mind, and your body to make sure those three aspects of your consciousness are accessible to guide your choices as your day unfolds.

Throughout your day, little conversations and adjustments would happen. As you emerged from your car, you would take a moment to shift your sense of pacing, from the rapid speed of travel to a more leisurely stroll that allows you to tune in to the trees and sunshine and get an energy snack from them. You would naturally notice when your body or mind has needs that do not match the demands of the moment. After half a lifetime of self-care, you would probably know how to automatically and gracefully listen, console, adjust, adapt, and reset your energies.

Because the language of energy is your source code, your first language, it will not take you years to gain fluency. Instead, you will awaken to ways you have already been using this language and build on those.

HOW TO USE THIS BOOK

Just as we learn language situationally, through interacting with native speakers, you can use this book in a number of ways:

First, just read it straight through as an immersion experience. Let the ideas and frameworks and stories filter in. Learn the language of energy the way you first learned language as an infant: taking in all the sounds and gradually making sense of what you are hearing, all the while constructing your own personal understanding of the world.

Second, use the book as an exploration guide, dipping in and out wherever you feel drawn. Many chapters offer a number of explorations, labeled "Play With It," that guide you in just playing with the concepts. With these, I often offer illustrative examples of my own experiences as I explored these ideas while writing this book.

Third, work your way systematically through the book, applying the concepts and exercises to your own life. The book is full of healing stories that illustrate different people's health challenges and approaches to wellness. These are coupled with energy exercises and meditations that provide specific tools.

Finally, throughout the book, the structure, syntax, vocabulary, and usage of the language of energy are linked to how we actually acquire language as children. This is not a foreign tongue to be learned by rote memorization and grammar drills. Instead, it is our baseline idiom that governs how we communicate within and with others. *The Language Your Body Speaks* will help you to evolve your awareness of the language of energy and your native ability to speak and understand it.

Chapter One

POWERFUL MEDICINE

Thinking Outside the Box about Healing

Mother Teresa was visiting a health center in India when she came across a man in extreme spasms. His arms, legs, and torso were all contorted and twisted, and he was in agony. She stepped up to him, took one look — a look I can only describe as pragmatic compassion — and then began stroking him all over his body, firmly and rhythmically. It was not a gentle stroke of consolation, as if to say, *There, there, oh suffering one.* It was more like the calls of a coxswain, bringing a crew into perfect synchronization. As she stroked, his body unfurled, released, relaxed, until he was lying there with arms and legs extended, in obvious release from the pain.

I saw this scene in a video years ago and have revisited the interaction repeatedly over the years, puzzling over just what I saw. On one level, it was the power of loving intention. But it was not just some special Mother Teresa healing magic. If it was a miracle, it was the miracle of the simple and ordinary: the power of touch, and someone's clear will and intention overriding whatever massive electrical mess was going on in that poor man's body.

Although Mother Teresa was a skilled healer, the powers she used in that moment were something that I — or anyone — could have called upon to help that suffering soul.

Mother Teresa had the tools for the job in her hands. And somehow, she also had the inner certainty about what to do in that moment and how to do it.

First, she believed she could make a difference. She saw a soul suffering in front of her and stepped forward to do something about it. She practiced a form of active compassion. She asked herself: *Is there something I can do for this man in this moment that might help? Can I respond to what the body and soul in front of me are expressing and asking for?*

Second, she used touch to communicate (using energy medicine rather than chemical interventions). She trusted her hands. She used them to communicate a focused, calm, organized rhythm to the man's body. The communication spoke directly to his body's energies, gave them the organization they needed, and overrode whatever misfires his nervous system was producing. Our hands emit energy that *speaks* to the energies that make up and run the body. She knew how to use her hands to carry out this communication.

Third, she had inner guidance on how to proceed. Call it faith, or years of habitual listening to her inner compass, but Mother Teresa needed only a few seconds to get a sense of what would be helpful in that situation. Her inner compass was well-calibrated through years of use in practical situations. She did not do a medical triage or logical analysis; she clearly consulted her own inner wisdom and came up with a response that was timely and appropriate. She was not moving from person to person indiscriminately stroking them all!

Fourth, she was willing to try something and observe the results. One of the big differences between Mother Teresa and other people wishing to help was that she stepped in and acted. She didn't pray over the man, tell him he created his own reality, or exhort him to change his diet. She didn't make an appointment, sign him up for ongoing care, or give him a treatment plan. She stepped in and tried something in the moment that she sensed he needed right then. In doing that, she came up with one key to help that man and the people around him understand what might support his healing over time. This is what we do each time we engage in energy dialogue.

Was it the complete answer to how to heal the illness that sent his body into spasms? Probably not, but it was a response that he didn't have before his encounter with Mother Teresa.

In self-healing, we too often lack those four elements: belief you can make a difference; energy medicine tools and conscious touch; inner guidance; and willingness to act in the moment to address what is in front of you. These form a foundation for using energy dialogue to heal yourself.

Mother Teresa's intervention wasn't medical, but it was powerful medicine. It was a direct communication in the moment. Can you imagine how different your life would be if, in each moment, you could respond to what is and provide something your body, mind, and spirit need right now?

• • • EXERCISE: MOTHER TERESA TOUCH • • •

This can be tried for nearly *any* ailment, except one in which it is painful to touch the skin or body. It is particularly good for muscle spasms, stomachaches, digestive woes, heart irregularities, mental irritation or upset, many autoimmune conditions, and even organic issues like kidney disease.

Using a regular rhythm, either one that matches a heartbeat *(lub-dub)* or one that is brisk but not too aggressive, stroke repeatedly on the body. You can imagine yourself as the coxswain of a rowing crew, helping all the rowers to synchronize their strokes and pull the boat forward in a strong but steady rhythm. It is helpful to stroke downward along the whole body, including the torso, arms, and legs, but you may find that stroking sideways or at angles is also helpful.

Stroking behind the ears and down the back of the head is great for calming reactivity. Stroking down the back and front helps you to ground.

Continue until you feel a release (if you are doing it on yourself) or until the person you are helping takes a deep breath or asks you to stop.

Experiment with how firmly to stroke. Get feedback from your own body, and if you are helping another, from that person. Too light a stroke may irritate the skin and body. You want the *rhythm*, *pace*, and *clarity* of the stroking to set a pattern to replace the confused discomfort or reactivity of the body.

Here is a suggested pattern to use:

Start with your head and stroke from front to back, crown to neck for four to eight counts.

Cross your arms and reach across to each shoulder with your hands, then stroke down both arms for four to eight counts.

Stroke down your front, from collarbone to the bottom of your torso, with one hand on each side of the midline, palms open and covering as much territory as possible. Do this rhythmically in counts of three, four, or five (experiment with what feels best), for as many repetitions as you need.

Starting at your upper chest, place both hands side by side at the midline, and spread the skin horizontally, stroking in counts of three, four, or five. Move your hands down the midline to your belly and repeat, then to your lower belly and repeat.

Stroke down both legs together if you can, or one at a time if that is easier. Stroke the fronts, the inner thighs and calves, the outer thighs and calves, and if you can reach them, the backs of your legs.

If you can get someone to help, have them stroke down your back. If no one is available, use a towel. First rub the towel over your heart to infuse it with caring energy, then pull it down your back.

•   •   •   •   •   •

QUESTIONING THE NORMS

In traditional cultures, medicine is an act, a substance, a symbolic object, or a ritual that catalyzes healing. The medicine man or woman acts as a healer, priest, educator, mediator, teacher, and power broker. In our conventional, allopathic context, taking medicine has come to mean pharmaceuticals, and the practice of medicine is primarily focused on diagnosing problems and attacking illness, not on cultivating harmony between mind, body, and spirit and catalyzing the body's abilities to heal.

We take so much for granted as natural and normal in our conventional medicine that would make no sense to someone from outside:

- Imagine touring a hospital with a shaman and explaining why we think it supports health to put people who are sick in bland, sterile rooms, apart from loved ones and beloved or sacred objects.
- Imagine taking your visitor to a medical office and trying to explain how the doctor can figure out in ten to twenty minutes what is making someone sick without examining the patient's life, relationships, food, living quarters, spiritual state, thoughts, energetic affiliations, or other key factors that are considered crucial in most healing traditions.
- Imagine touring a pharmaceutical company with a tribal herbalist and explaining how little white items with no obvious link to nature — or spirit — can serve as medicines.

Allopathic medicine, when it works, can be spectacular. When it doesn't work, it can get the whole process of healing spectacularly wrong.

I had a friend from elementary school who was diagnosed at the age of twenty with a rare kind of cancer. The whole process of finding and diagnosing his disease was a story of unlikely successes: This was not a cancer with many symptoms (he had a lump near one of his testicles); the blood work he got was not routine, but for some reason his particular insurance allowed the doctor to order it; and the specialist who examined him happened to practice in a teaching hospital where an eager intern thought to test for this nearly unheard-of cancer. And although my friend was given less than a one percent chance of survival, he did survive. They were just pioneering a trial of a new treatment and were able to include him in the study. He was one of the lucky ones for whom it worked.

If the story ended there, you could call this a spectacular triumph of allopathic medicine.

But our shaman visitor might have some follow-up questions. Was my friend healed or merely cancer-free? Had the circumstances that caused his body to go out of balance and develop the cancer been addressed? Was he able to heal his spirit and pursue his soul's true path into a fulfilling life? Could he reintegrate into harmony with people and community? Did he find a new balance that allowed him to live life in a healthier way?

We don't expect doctors to ask these questions. Their follow-up is generally designed to identify whether the cancer is now in remission and to make sure there is no recurrence. In our culture, it is the purview of psychologists, ministers, nutritionists, complementary medicine practitioners, and even family members to deal with further aspects of healing (if we even realize these actually are aspects of healing). Of course, ideally, it would also be part of each person's self-care.

In fact, my friend never found wellness. For a while, he was happy and relieved to be cancer-free. But the instability in his systems, which had triggered the cancer, was still there, and it took many forms over the next twenty-five years of his life.

Although he had regular checkups, the focus was so much on ruling out a return of the cancer that he developed a number of issues that were not treated as skillfully. His thyroid fluctuated from overactive to underactive. He married, but his unaddressed mood problems finally caused his marriage to rupture. He began to withdraw from life in ways that became apparent in retrospect, but at the time were masked by the melancholy, aches, and pains caused by the medications and divorce. And at the age of forty-five, he committed suicide.

This is not a condemnation of allopathic medicine! In my friend's situation, allopathic medicine did what it is designed to do and produced better results than studies might have predicted. This is a commentary on how we, as a culture, view healing, wellness, and the relationships between body, mind, and spirit.

The purpose of this discussion is not to bash our Western system of medicine and healing, but I think it is important to occasionally remind ourselves, as users of that system, about the crisis in health care we are experiencing in the United States and other industrialized countries. The training, technology, and delivery of allopathic medicine is so unwieldy, true healing frequently gets lost.

What is most relevant in calling out the health care *crisis* is that it pushes us to go back to the drawing board and rethink healing, health, care, and how to understand illness and wellness. Maybe most important for this book on self-healing using energy medicine, it pushes us to rethink our roles as participants in our own well-being.

Speaking Allopathy

allopathic: *relating to or being a system of medicine that aims to combat disease by using remedies (such as drugs or surgery) which produce effects that are different from or incompatible with those of the disease being treated.*

— *Merriam-Webster's Dictionary*

Western medical systems are built on the foundations of science and the scientific model: That is the language, the mindset, we turn to when we want to influence the body. There are plusses and minuses to this. There are medical interventions that succeed in ways that other systems of healing might not: A surgery to repair a ruptured organ can be a lifesaver. However, if you want to learn to participate in your own healing, science is probably not the best model — or language — for you to use.

Consider the predominant medical perspective for a moment. It sees you as a primarily physical organism, animated via multiple chemical and organic processes. The workings of your body are perceived as a complex of interconnected functional systems. And when something goes wrong, the interventions tend to focus on altering chemical communications via pharmaceuticals, conducting surgical fixes to repair the physical structures, and bombarding *invaders* — such as germs, viruses, bacteria, and even your own rogue cells — using toxins such as chemotherapy, hoping these will kill the invaders but not the body hosting them.

This perspective has its limitations for me as a self-healer.

If I see myself as a set of interacting chemical processes, I am dependent on scientists to study the right things and to come up with the right interventions. I have to accept the pharmaceuticals that come with pages of side effects because I believe in the interventions those chemicals can bring. Yet the holes in our scientific knowledge base are extensive, starting with who participated in the research and who funded what trials. In addition, although the belief is that your body communicates via hormones, hormone specialists will tell you that they know amazingly little about what these agents are and exactly how they work.

If I think of myself primarily in scientific terms, then unless I can learn all the complexities and lingo, I am dependent on experts to help me understand my own body and, for that matter, my own mind. I don't ask my body what it wants or needs because I don't expect to understand the answers. And I most likely won't listen to the answers until they have been scientifically validated.

If I believe that healing is a matter of balancing the chemistry, then I can find myself with expensive bottles of pills and tinctures trying desperately to modify chemical communications that are far more subtle than the pills can truly regulate. What if I need half a dose one day, a triple dose the next, and no dose the day after that? What if I need the chemical supplement at 10 AM, but at 3 PM the presence of that same chemical communication agent in my system is befuddling normal functions?

If I see my health challenges as arising exclusively from organic and chemical processes, then where do emotion, meaning, spirit, my behaviors, my beliefs, and lived experience fit in?

If I buy into the model of attacking disease, what do I do if the disease arises from lacks or imbalances in how I'm caring for my instrument? What do I do if the very agents meant to silence the symptoms or kill off the invaders interfere with my body's ability to maintain wellness?

If I buy into the mindset that sees my body as a machine, and illness as a malfunction of that machine, then I think in terms of very mechanistic fixes when something goes wrong, and I miss the communications about what my body, spirit, and mind are asking me to cultivate.

Speaking Energy

On the other hand, if I shift my perspective, and see myself as a web of energies, moving in patterns, creating my body in interaction with my mind (consciousness) and spirit, in a rich language that has *meaning*, then I can learn to tune in to those energies and patterns. I can learn to communicate with them in both specific and universal ways and create the conditions that allow my body and mind to thrive.

If I understand that my body is part of an energetic spectrum that spans spirit, mind, and body, then I will know that something going wrong with my body can be effectively addressed by working with that whole spectrum.

The language of energy is not a metaphor! It is as real as science as a way of understanding how we are constructed, and it offers us significant tools for interacting with our own being to support healing, health, well-being, and the creation of a meaningful life.

When you shift your perspective to understand the workings of your body, mind, and spirit as energy communications, healing becomes a very individualized and personal matter. And you don't have to learn Latin and study science to understand your instrument.

The capacity to understand — and speak — the language of energy is coded into us, every bit as much as the capacity to learn English or Chinese. But like learning English or Chinese, we need to be supported in learning to speak. We need to be exposed to the language of energy in its specifics to activate our innate ability to use it.

Your body is made of energy and communicates energetically. Even chemical communications, at their root, are energetic exchanges of protons and neutrons. Learning the language of energy gives you power to understand and shift the course of illness and disease. More important, it allows you not only to decode illness but also to encode wellness, since it works through interaction and dialogue with the energies that are moving and shifting within you, creating your physical, mental, and spiritual experience.

Speaking energy goes way beyond explaining physical phenomena using what science has discovered about the subtle energies. Speaking energy entails shifting how you understand yourself to be constructed and learning how to participate more consciously in the energetic exchanges within and around you. Practicing energy medicine similarly goes well beyond learning techniques or studying modalities. It involves activating your ability to speak the language of energy and addressing your body, mind, and spirit in their own native idiom.

However, using allopathic medicine or energy medicine does not need to be an either/or proposition when you are trying to address your health. There are times when allopathic medicine is a godsend, and times when energy medicine is a more effective mode of communication. Often, the two can complement each other.

My friend with the rare cancer got treated medically for cancer and that threat to his life was neutralized. But if he had been seen by his medical team as a web of meaningful exchanges that had fallen out of balance, creating cells that no longer followed healthy replication patterns, his practitioners might have addressed both the cellular issues *and* the imbalance in his web of meaning. He might have learned self-care tools that no practitioner can provide day in and day out. He might have found practices that balanced his body's chemistry from within. And he might have found true recovery and wellness, rather than cancer remission among his life-hampering imbalance.

A BROADER PERSPECTIVE ON HEALING

What does it mean to transcend the limitations of allopathic medicine and our shared cultural beliefs about healing? Too often when we are looking for new approaches, we turn to complementary medicine but bring our conventional medicine mindset to the task. We want the same old model of diagnosing problems, receiving treatment, and then taking a substance to medicate. We want approaches that are scientifically validated. How can you transcend these cultural expectations and learn to think differently in order to harness the true potential of energy healing?

Reclaim Subjectivity

The scientific mindset calls for objectivity and discourages subjectivity. This means that all the information that arises within you — your inner knowing, your experiential insights, your personal experience, the personal storyline in which the health challenge developed — is considered mostly irrelevant.

A young doctor finishing up her residency recently told me that she is not able to use her intuition in her job. She is expected to practice evidence-based medicine, which means she must cite studies that validate her medical choices. This might be a good idea if studies were funded to research all kinds of people and if these studies were able to account for the multiple dimensions of how disease and illness play out. But that isn't what happens.

By asking doctors to turn off their intuition and rely on evidence, I believe the medical profession is hampering the way the mind is designed to work: Right-brain intuition guides our journey, and left-brain logic works out the details of the itinerary. What would happen to medical care if doctors were encouraged to use both evidence *and* intuition to guide their choices, and they could use both medical and alternative remedies as needed?

Validate Your Authority to Determine Your Own Well-being

Related to the notion of subjectivity is the question of who has the authority to decide what you should do in order to heal — or even what healing would look like for you. In our culture, doctors are often seen as all-knowing priests, and friends and family tell us not to question that. Physicians' input can be valuable, but many of them don't distinguish well between what they know and don't know. Missing from their knowledge base is what your individual soul is trying to enact, how your lifestyle and beliefs affect your health, and how your energies — which underlie the chemical behaviors of your body — flow and interact.

The authority we give doctors and scientists to define our individual and collective truth is sometimes taken to an extreme. The other day I read an article with the teaser: "Scientists have proven the existence of past lives." The need to have something proven by science that has been explored and validated as a truth within many spiritual traditions is almost a caricature of our culture's obsession with scientific "proof." How can we trust ourselves to find our own path to healing when people around us are trained to ask: *Can that be proven scientifically? Has that been validated with medical tests? Is that what your doctor thinks?*

In this book, I use subjective information to guide the discussion as much as possible: I prefer using anecdotes that illuminate concepts and understandings rather than offering scientific studies to prove my points. This is a nonscientific form of discourse. You might ask yourself whether it bothers you to not have science repeatedly cited as an authority. Can what I am saying be true if I don't cite some study that proves it? I am not saying science is always wrong, nor am I rejecting science. Instead, I think focusing solely on science deflects us from understanding the communications of our bodies and minds. It undermines our confidence in our ability to participate in our own healing and it curtails other ways of knowing.

Be Willing to Be an Exception to the Rule

Allopathic medicine is based on studies that prove statistically that something is true or effective. A medication or treatment must work for a given percentage of people studied before it is approved for use, though sometimes the demonstrated effectiveness of a medication is not much greater than its placebo effect! There are good reasons for insisting a medication work for many, but this shuts out usages that might help individuals. Herbalists believe individualized potions are more effective than just giving the same generic treatment to everyone with the same complaint.

Years ago, in the early days of the AIDS epidemic, I had a client who told me he had healed his AIDS. He had been tested (a number of times) as HIV positive, and then he caught pneumonia, which bumped his diagnosis to active AIDS. After he recovered from the pneumonia, he worked on his health using spiritual and nutritional approaches, and after eight years, he was consistently testing HIV negative. I was amazed and excited to hear his story. I asked: "What do your doctors say? Have you shared your story with others?" The belief at that time was that AIDS could not be survived, much less healed.

He said he was choosing to keep his story private, explaining, "When I tell people, they either don't believe me or they believe I am in denial and will soon die. I have chosen *not* to live with their beliefs because that will overwhelm my own truth. So although I do occasionally get retested, I do not choose to live as an AIDS patient."

This man was an exception, and life is full of splendid, amazing exceptions from whom we have much to learn. What he taught me was not to discount individual solutions or exceptions to the rule. I also learned to be more aware of the power of social beliefs in healing.

If everyone around you believes you can't heal, it takes tremendous self-confidence and precious resources to break through that field of expectation to find your own path and truth, to become the exception to the rule.

Sue was a nurse who came to see me at the strong request of her partner, who believed in complementary medicine. Sue did not. But since she was scheduled to undergo a procedure the next day to have her thyroid irradiated (which essentially kills the nonfunctioning thyroid so they can balance your thyroid function through pills), she decided to give energy healing a try. I agreed to see her on the condition that, afterward, she have her thyroid blood levels retested before she went ahead with the planned medical procedure.

She agreed. When I tuned in to her throat energetically, I found that her thyroid had basically switched off. I used the language of energy to dialogue with her thyroid and move the switches to the on position. I could see the glandular tissue reanimate and return to normal functioning. I could hear it, the way you hear a refrigerator start up once you change the fuse that has blown a circuit.

She had gone off all thyroid medication in anticipation of the surgery and felt wiped out without it. Within a few minutes of resetting the switches, she reported (with some surprise) that she felt normal again. Joking, she asked, "Did you slip me a thyroid pill?" In a way I did. I activated the communication system of her energies to reanimate the gland, which in turn produced what her body needed!

The next day, Sue followed through on her promise and asked her doctor to test her thyroid levels one more time. The blood work came back showing normal on all parameters. The doctor was mystified. He asked her what she had done and whether she had somehow taken some thyroid medication, though he knew as a nurse she knew better. She told him about our session.

He barely let her get the words "energy healer" out of her mouth before hurrying to assure her that "idiopathic recovery" occasionally happened and telling her he was canceling her surgery. He asked her to return in a week to see if her levels were still adequate and her thyroid was still functioning. (It was.) What he didn't do was show any interest or curiosity about her unique experience. He didn't want to know more about energy healing or what led her to try it. He didn't care that this individual had found a solution that might hold promise for other individuals. He had a name for what happened — *idiopathic* means unique to the individual — and therefore, it was not valid or interesting to him.

I have seen this response again and again as clients who experienced successful healing or self-healing encountered disbelief or dismissal from doctors, family, friends, and even within themselves. So I have come to see the wisdom of my ex-AIDS client who wanted to fly beneath the social radar. Using energy medicine successfully includes being willing to be an exception, to beat the odds, to defy gravity, to celebrate the unique capacities of our own bodies and energy systems. It is important to leave room for miracles in each dialogue we have with our own physical being. Experience has taught me that what is sometimes seen as a miracle is in fact just a matter of knowing how to communicate via energy.

Learn to Cultivate Evidence from Multiple Realms

I once accompanied a seventy-three-year-old friend with stage IV breast cancer through her medical experience. When she was diagnosed, the nurse said: "Now you'll get the million-dollar treatment." She was sent for test after test, shuffling from doctor to doctor, and found herself in a kind of cancer world where natives knew the routine and she was whirled from one invasive experience to another.

My friend wanted to participate in her own healing. She also wanted to know the scientific basis of the recommendations for the myriad decisions she needed to make. At each decision point, she would ask: "What do the studies say about this?" And after evasions and assurances that her doctors were recommending the best practice, she would ultimately discover they didn't really know. The research was based on young women or not disaggregated for other key factors, like lifestyle or nutrition. The science just wasn't there. And the "standard of care" recommendations were not based on women her age or with her self-care skills. They were essentially *guesses*, albeit educated guesses, masquerading as science.

At one point, my friend had to make the harrowing decision to reject further medical intervention, without the benefit of any relevant scientific evidence and against the standardized recommendations of her doctors. She chose to use the evidence of her body, and her own intuition and wisdom, to make her choice.

That risk paid off: She has remained cancer-free for five years. But the process was agonizing. And she had to give up the notion that science was the only source of evidence that could guide her to figure out what was best for her *as an individual.*

While more and better research would help, that won't solve the basic problem. The scientific method calls for controlled environments in which to study a phenomenon and find the truth. But life isn't lived in isolated circumstances, and studying something in a controlled, laboratory setting often alters its behavior. How can researchers possibly control all the variables to study how a particular body will respond when it has gone out of balance and developed a particular disease? Often, research studies give us the illusion that we understand phenomena when we don't.

Instead, it makes more sense to incorporate additional ways of assessing and knowing what a particular mind-body-spirit is undergoing. It also makes sense to incorporate nutritional supports, lifestyle, and energy medicine — wellness practices — into the mix.

The Western medical system favors information gleaned from isolating things to understand them, while sometimes dismissing the wisdom of understanding your health in the context of who you are, how you live, what kind of nourishment you receive, how well your instrument is played, what role your mind plays, what your soul's purpose might be, and how environments have influenced you historically and in the present. These dimensions are significant in energy medicine.

As a self-healer, it is important that you cultivate and assess evidence of what your body needs, can tolerate, and is expressing. That evidence might have some relevant science to bolster it. But it may also be subjective, arising from dialoguing with your body in various contexts and situations. It will be informed by your history and illuminated by alternative expertise about how mind, body, and spirit can heal.

The notion that we should defer to scientific understandings, laboratory results, and standardized treatments even when our own experience is telling us otherwise runs deep in our culture. As a self-healer, you may find it more effective to treat yourself as the main character in a novel, dealing with a rich plot, setting, and cast of characters all influencing your evolution, rather than trying to isolate your symptoms and assess your situation scientifically.

Recognize Your Illness as a Falling Away from Wellness

In allopathic medicine, gallbladder disease is studied as a phenomenon that happens to the gallbladder as an organ. The literature on gallbladder disease focuses on how the organ behaves under various conditions and what can be done to alter that. It does not usually focus on what happened in each patient's life, what behaviors, physiology, and energy usage caused their gallbladder to tank. Ten patients with gallbladder disease might receive somewhat individualized approaches, but basically the doctor is treating their gallbladder.

In Chinese medicine (and most other forms of energy medicine), a diseased gallbladder is seen more as the result of imbalance in the whole energetic circulation of the individual. Ten people who have diseased gallbladders are treated as ten different energy profiles. Disease is seen as a falling away from wellness (not as a separate thing), so the path to wellness for each individual has to do with what kind of person they are and what is happening for them in terms of nutrition, energy flows, their environmental and lifestyle choices, and more.

This is more than just saying allopathic medicine treats the illness whereas energy medicine works with the person experiencing the illness. In our culture, we tend to think of illness as something apart from life and from the individual experiencing the illness. We medicalize life processes such as childbirth and death, and within the medical context, we get depersonalized. An extreme example of this is when hospital personnel refer to someone as "the heart attack in room C320." It is a reflection of society's philosophy about where illness and wellness reside.

If I believe my illness is something I caught, or some faulty part that has malfunctioned, or something only a specialist can address, then I must wait for the drugs, surgeon, or specialist to come rescue me. But if I believe my illness is part of how I function, then I can shift my functioning and nudge my body toward wellness.

If I believe my symptoms are a personal indicator of my internal communications, and not just a named disease with prescribed treatment protocols, then I can dialogue with my body to change the conversation and often heal it from within. Even if my gallbladder must be removed because the imbalance has stressed the organ into nonviability, I still need to improve the conversation and address the whole-self imbalances that led to the organ failure.

Try this: When you are grappling with a named disease or condition, ask yourself how having this condition serves you. Then ask yourself what *ease* would entail and how you could cultivate that.

Affirm the Unique Qualities You Embody

If you go to a dog show, you can see a huge variety of breeds, each massively different, and yet each is called a dog. If you go to the pound, you can expand on this variety. There are commonalities among all dogs, but you would never take care of or medicate a greyhound the same way you would a Saint Bernard or a Chihuahua.

Somehow, when it comes to healing, our culture seems to think a body is a body is a body. Maybe you will require a bit more or less medicine than the next person, based on your size, age, and gender (though even those distinctions are often ignored). But basically, we see the human body as more similar than different.

Donna Eden, an energy medicine pioneer who can see the body's subtle energies, says frequently that, although there are common patterns (chakras, meridians, the aura, and other energy systems), "each person's energies are as unique as a thumbprint."

Can you imagine working with a healing practitioner who helped you identify what can support your individual moving dynamic of energies to thrive?

This is a very different approach than our medical mentality of asking: *What is wrong and how can we fix it?* Allopathic medicine assumes that a blood profile is usually sufficient to understand what is happening, ignoring the fact that even the time lapse between the tests and the consultation brings a change.

What if we understood the body as an ongoing story, with multiple plotlines weaving in and out? What if instead of looking to eradicate what is wrong, we focused on bringing those plotlines into greater clarity, harmony, and balance?

The notion of sameness makes us miss crucial cues in healing and self-healing. It keeps us from understanding our own breed and individuality and measuring our expectations against that. For example, if your natural energy is slow and stately (like a tortoise), then trying to keep up in a world full of hares will cause you stress and eventually illness.

Knowing what *kind* of person you are is key to self-healing. Knowing what your soul's purpose is, what energizes or drains you personally and specifically, what particular foods are nourishing to you, is part of being able to heal. Yet this conversation rarely comes up in allopathic contexts. We may be told to lower our stress, but each individual has a very different relationship to stress. What stresses me may make your heart sing. Recognizing individuality is crucial if we don't want to jump from one set of *shoulds* to another.

The idea of measuring ourselves against a norm is deeply ingrained in us. It affects how we interpret our health and success. If you can suspend your socialized mind enough to see yourself not as a body (species human, subtype female or male) and instead see yourself as a web of energies, a web of *meaning*, you can see how medicine that is individualized to your unique web would be more effective than something designed to manipulate the chemistry of a generic physical body.

Understand the Interplay between Body, Mind, and Spirit

Early anatomists dissected corpses to understand the organs and workings of the body. This evolved into a practice of medicine that is still focused on the body as an object, apart from whatever might animate it. The cosmology behind this suggests a separation between the physical, emotional, and spiritual dimensions of our being. Allopathic doctors are not trained to deal with our emotional or spiritual health. This is problematic if you believe your body, mind, and spirit are interrelated.

On the other hand, cultures that have developed highly evolved forms of energy medicine (China, India, Tibet, aboriginal, and so on) evolved out of a cosmology that considers the mental, spiritual, and physical realms to be interrelated. Practitioners use observation and experimentation, herbs (chemistry), and physical manipulations, just as Western medicine does, but they also use intuition and expanded mental abilities to glean information.

Insights into the health of the body are developed in the larger context of who you are. Evidence is gathered from the patient, the family or tribe, the body's behavior, movements of the subtle energies, and elemental factors based on the group's spiritual understandings of how we are constructed. In most cases, healers look at what is needed not only on the physical level but also on the level of soul and mind.

Yoga practitioners do not just identify weak muscles and do exercises to strengthen them; they work to build strength throughout the body, mind, and spirit.

This is more than preventive medicine — it is *proactive medicine,* or practices that promote wellness.

Understanding about how the soul constructs the body, and how the body reacts to mental and spiritual conditions, is part of most energy healing traditions. But it is often mocked and discredited in allopathic contexts and may be discredited by your friends and family if they see the allopathic model as exclusively valid. It may be seen as superstition or guesswork, primitive or ignorant of reality (as defined in our rationalist, scientific culture). If we want to develop a contemporary understanding of self-healing using energy medicine, we need to recognize this. Social prejudice against complementary healing has diminished greatly in the past twenty years. But it is still alive and kicking in many settings.

As you set out to learn the language of energy, I invite you to keep your outsider perspective handy, to explore and experiment, to try things on for size, to tune in and investigate what feels true for you. It is not necessary to reject allopathic medicine to learn self-healing through energy medicine. But it *is* necessary to be willing to work from the inside out, determining for yourself how you are constructed, how to dialogue with and bolster your own unique thumbprint of energies, and what energy nourishment would best support your journey in this life.

• • • MEDITATION: EXPLORING THE WEB OF MEANING • • •

Read these instructions into a recorder or ask a friend to read this slowly for you:

Shut your eyes for a moment and tune in to your body as a creature, like a dog or cat. You may even want to give yourself a good rub, as you would your family pet. Wag your tail. Flex each foot and feel it as you set it down again. Stretch and bend the fingers of each hand, feeling how intricate and amazing your hands are. Shift your back in a swaying motion side to side, feeling how your spine can flex and bend. Feel the flesh, muscle, sinew, bones, and organs that make up this miraculous instrument.

I call this creature your *Earth Elemental Self*. It feels solid, but each organ, bone, and connector is a community of cells, which are in their turn small energy generators made of molecules and atoms, communicating endlessly within themselves and with other cells to collectively create this thing we call a body.

Now, tune in to your mind: the knowing, thinking part of you, the *Talking Self*. If your attention is up in your head, in your brain, let that awareness of mind expand to include the knowing, the *me*, that fills your whole body. Feel into your heart area and its wisdom, your solar plexus, your gut, your hands and feet. Let your awareness travel wherever this Talking Self resides. Your Talking Self isn't limited to your body space. You can send your mind out into other situations, other places, using your imagination. Feel this part of you that creates dramas, develops your identity and life story, codifies experience using language, thought, and perception. This self is also made of energies, more subtle perhaps than the energies that compose matter.

Now, tune in to your *Wiser Self*. Feel into your soul, or Source Self. Does it take a form, have sound, color, sensation, light, or come into your awareness through direct knowing? Is your Wiser Self standing apart from you, or is it cohabiting the same area as your body? Is your Wiser Self alone or standing with others? Your Wiser Self is also made of energy — perhaps the most obviously energetic of the three selves. How do you perceive those energies?

The life-force energy you are made of is not neutral; it has light, color, vibration, movement, pattern, and *meaning*. Just as each note in the musical scale comes together into songs that communicate to us, the energies that you are made of aggregate and communicate meaning. Feel all that meaning that creates you. Let yourself feel the web of energies, spanning a spectrum from spirit through mind through body, moving and exchanging and communicating and pulsing with life.

This pulsing field of meaning is *you*: a web of energies communicating and connecting, forming patterns and working independently. You are a web of meaning. Feel that, as you felt your own physical body at the start of this exercise. When you are ready, open your eyes, and look at everything in the world around you as interacting energies your instrument has learned to perceive, then interpret, as form, thought, or spirit.

• • • • • •

PRACTICE TIPS

- Adopt an energy medicine mindset, like putting on a pair of outsider glasses, to get a handle on what is happening in your body, mind, and spirit. What might your situation look like to an alien, recently landed? What tools do you have — from language, from literature, from life, from friends and teachers — that allow you to understand what is happening for you now?

- Try using nonscientific language to describe your situation. Metaphors are great: "I feel like a volcano about to erupt." "I feel like a mouse being toyed with by a cat." "My body feels angry and rebellious — like a teen trying to find her own identity." Be subjective in characterizing what is going on for you.

- Spend time gathering and assessing evidence of what your body needs, can tolerate, and is expressing. Put aside what you have read about nutrition, body chemistry, even spirituality, and just see what your own body wants to tell you. Treat yourself as an infant who can't yet talk but who can still express wants and needs. (I provide more guidance on how to engage in energy dialogue in later chapters.)

- Try the "Mother Teresa Touch" (page 15) on yourself when you are feeling emotional, physical, or social imbalance. What are you hearing/understanding about your situation as you do it, and what are you communicating?

- Explore any illness or imbalance in relation to how you function. What is the story that gives it context? For example, I recently caught a cold that everyone around me was getting. It is valid to just say "a cold is a cold." But in my specific case, I caught it after three months of high stress. It hit my throat at a time when communications were particularly challenged for me. It didn't affect my lungs, but it hung on and on, sapping my energy to move forward. What can these conditions teach me about how I need to adjust my functioning and nudge my body toward wellness? What needs did the cold meet (albeit in an unlovely way)? Even though everyone I knew was responding to the virus, what did my particular cold have to offer me in my creation of a life, relationships, plotline, and body?

Chapter Two

DIVING INTO THE
LANGUAGE OF ENERGY

Language is more than just words and sentence structure. It embraces all the ways you codify your experience and how you exchange with others. Similarly, healing is more than just finding techniques to fix what is wrong. Using the language of energy to heal includes finding ways to address and shift how you experience and interact with life.

Some years ago I was captivated by the film *Arrival*, starring Amy Adams, which really brought this concept of language home to me. In the film, Adams plays a linguistics professor recruited by the army to figure out how to communicate with an alien spacecraft, one of twelve encircling the globe. Adams is in a race against time to discover who these beings are and what their intentions toward the planet might be.

The bulk of the film shows how a linguist can figure out the workings of a language (and whether a language even exists) when the speakers don't use sound, words, or other linguistic building blocks we are familiar with. In the case of these beings — spoiler alert — Adams comes to realize that they communicate by emitting smoke-like glyphs, a kind of bar-code language, in conjunction with telepathy: mind-to-mind shaping of experience and concepts.

Most fascinating to me was that the film does not stop with the linguistic triumph of cracking the code of the language. It shows how Adams's character learns to understand the mindset of these visitors — their conceptions of time, space, and connection — that make them clearly kindred spirits. The film is not about learning vocabulary and grammar. It is about communication itself — finding shared expression, dialoguing, expressing meaning (the aliens need help to save their world) — and about the relationships that form when communication is successful.

Each time you enter into energy dialogue with yourself, you are investigating what your body, spirit, and mind are trying to express in a multidimensional language that is not composed of words and sentences. Through this dialogue, you are building a deeper, more-engaged relationship with yourself.

Sylvia, who was diagnosed with two kinds of metastatic stage IV cancer, had a similarly urgent mission to learn how to communicate with a body that was screaming at her in life-and-death terms. She needed to learn the language of energy and to dialogue with her body, spirit, and mind in order to figure out what would save her planet.

A hard worker who gave selflessly to her many children and grandchildren, Sylvia kept a family business going and was the glue holding a whole extended family together. As great as she was at caring for others, her selflessness took its toll on her body. She sought medical care too late and was not a candidate for chemo. Essentially, she was sent home to die.

Because the diagnosis was so severe, it liberated her to think outside the box. She decided that whether she was going to live or die, she would make each moment count. She would listen to her body and let it guide her and teach her each moment she had left. Using what she knew from parenting preverbal infants, she tuned in over and over again to perceive what her body wanted, needed, and was trying to communicate.

Her focus was not to delay death but to catch hold of life.

Sylvia learned simple energy medicine techniques to get her energies circulating and interacting more effectively. She engaged in an hour-by-hour experiment to recognize what her energies were asking of her, rather than following a preprogrammed cancer protocol. She listened to what foods spoke to her, and she brought in more life force via fruits, vegetables, and juicing. She experimented with other nutritional supports that showed up on her radar in synchronous ways.

Most important for her self-healing journey, she focused her ability to care for others onto herself, reassessing what mattered to her, letting go of all agendas except for dialoguing with her body, taking in the love her family gave her, letting go of needing to be the glue for her family, and deepening her spiritual practice.

A year later, she was pronounced cancer-free.

Sylvia didn't discover some formula for using energy medicine (or nutrition and spiritual inputs) to heal cancer, since it wasn't cancer that got healed: It was Sylvia. The cancer was a very loud shout from her body saying something had gone wrong in her body-mind-spirit communications. The path to healing was how Sylvia dialogued with her energies, supporting her three selves to draw in the behaviors, substances, and healthier storyline that allowed her immune system to find a new normal.

Your body has the inbuilt ability to heal, to adapt, and to function under diverse circumstances. No one else heals it: not the doctor, the shaman, the energy healer, the beloved, or the medication. When we heal, we are not attacking disease; we are finding ease. We are not eradicating illness; we are redefining wellness and living it. We are not just seeking absence of pain or symptoms; we are listening to and responding to the pain and symptoms in recognition of what they are communicating. This is what Sylvia's body taught her.

Pain and symptoms are messengers. The goal, before we sedate or mute them, is to receive the message, thank the messenger sincerely, and then offer that messenger what comfort is possible within the context of responding to the messages.

Cultivating wellness moment by moment will support the body's amazing ability to heal. Here are some major keys to self-healing you might find helpful:

- Come back to the breath.
- Step into the *now.*
- Engage in authentic dialogue with your energies.
- Affirm core truths.

- Make space for your body to heal.
- Choose actions, thoughts, and environments that support well-being.

This can't happen if we are busy blah-blah-blahing to the body with chemicals, blasting it with complex and expensive treatments, expecting practitioners to do all the work, and buying into disease models that the body can't understand. The body understands wellness. When it falls away from that, the key to self-healing is to get creative in finding ways to guide it back home!

FIRST LANGUAGE

Like the language used by the aliens in *Arrival*, the language your body speaks is much more complex, dynamic, and multidimensional than merely sounds organized into words, arrayed in sentences and paragraphs. If you have ever been blessed to be around infants and watched them engage with the world around them — learning sounds and gestures and how to communicate their needs — you have a baseline familiarity with this first language.

Right from the start, infants have ways of communicating. They don't say, "Please pass me a new diaper"! They wriggle, shift their breathing, or turn red and wail. They look around or fix their gaze. They turn toward the loving arms that are holding them, or they stretch and go rigid and struggle to move away. Any experienced parent will tell you that infants are each unique in temperament and in how they communicate. That is part of the fun (and frustration) of parenting. What is going on for these little beings, newly arrived? Who are they, and how can we communicate with them? How can we soothe, nourish, love, protect, teach, and stimulate them and speak their language?

When you were an infant, long before you learned your native tongue, you were activating the language of energy. You vocalized, babbled, and explored sounds that communicate and move energy. Researchers believe that babies babble sounds from every known language, only gradually reducing their range as some sounds get reinforced by people around them and others receive no echo or response.

Your infant self did the equivalent with your physical being and evolving mind: You touched, tasted, felt, looked at, listened to, smelled, and attuned with objects, people, and energies. You explored both your instrument and the world around you using movement, gesture, facial expressions, and all your senses.

You also perceived and communicated energetically. You knew instinctively even then how to react to unspoken tension, to differentiate between heavy silence and calm loving silence, and to recognize authentic attention versus rote action on the part of your caregivers.

Most infants can see or otherwise perceive energies. We recognize that in some ways. We say: "Little Michael really reacts when his dad is stressed," or "Alethia is comfortable with some strangers and not others."

Because many of us in Western culture don't tend to believe ourselves capable of directly perceiving subtle energies or of telepathic, energetic communications, we dismiss the uncanny stares, unexplained responses, and prescient comments made by young children as imagination. Over time, most children learn to filter out their inborn abilities to perceive energies in favor of perceiving what the shared belief systems will affirm.

SENSORIMOTOR

Developmental psychologists call the first two years of life the *sensorimotor* stage. It is our time to explore, investigate, experiment, sense, and discover our instrument and build up an understanding of the world around us. This understanding is as much a part of the language of energy as the particular words we eventually learn to speak. If I have no experience with a ball, then I can learn that word in several languages and still not understand it. If, on the other hand, I have direct experience with a ball — I have felt it, smelled it, tasted it, rolled it, banged it, and so on — then that becomes my energetic baseline understanding.

Like many people, you may find that this early phase of learning concepts was also fraught with learning fear, caution, negative blowback, dismissal, stress, or restriction, depending on what was going on in your childhood home. The body chemistry that arose from that energetic learning is coded into your mind and nervous system and creates a level of stress that your logical mind can't calm with thought or words.

Your energies need direct energetic communication — tapping, stroking, crooning, bathing in a soothing color, sound, shape, gesture, or smell — in order to calm.

Your healing may require a return to a sensorimotor style of interacting with the world.

You may need to be willing to return to direct encounters with energies and to build up new, cleaner concepts of the world on a visceral level, piece by piece. Illnesses arise from accumulated stresses if, as a child, you learned a baseline distrust of the physical world, other people, or your ability to perceive a situation and respond appropriately.

Maralies was a grandchild of a Holocaust survivor. Her mother's mother, Elsa, spent a number of years in a concentration camp as a young girl (Maralies never knew many details), and she married one of the American soldiers who helped to liberate the camp. Elsa moved to the United States and did her best to put her life in Germany behind her. She embraced American culture to an almost exaggerated degree. Maralies's mother, Bettina, described Elsa as a terrified-perfectionist-Betty-Crocker-wannabe.

Money was tight, but Elsa and her husband scrimped and saved so Bettina could go to college. Bettina and her husband were both lawyers, and Maralies felt she grew up with almost too much support: She had music lessons, art lessons, math tutoring, and expectations that she would engage in sports, get great grades, and basically perform well in everything. Maralies *was* very accomplished. But she described life growing up with her own mother as never being enough. Every achievement was a prelude to the next great achievement. There was always this sense of the unseen enemy or danger and the fear of a misstep, which was probably passed down to her from her grandmother Elsa.

When I met Maralies, she had a diagnosis of Crohn's disease and a tentative diagnosis of lupus. She had turned her considerable talents to figuring out how to manage her diet, exercise, rest, activity, and every other aspect of her life to keep her symptoms at bay. She wanted to see if energy medicine could clear the Crohn's and lupus from her energy field. She was treading water with her management plan and felt exhausted from constant vigilance.

I spent a few moments feeling my way into Maralies's energies, and I realized that I was communicating with a being who was on constant red alert. Although Maralies seemed calm on the surface and seemed to be practicing excellent self-care, underneath was a siren going *WAAAH WAAAH WAAAH* every time we discussed what she was doing for herself. It was as if I was dealing with an unheard infant, wailing because no one was responding to her cries.

I asked her about that sense of an inner alarm, and her grandmother Elsa's story emerged. She said: "I feel like I am somehow still reacting to her experiences, even though I never even heard details!"

We talked about this and experimented a bit. We interacted with several of her energy systems using energy testing and found they were disorganized. Then I handed her a teddy bear to hug. She hugged it, and several of the energy systems we had pre-tested now had become organized. I asked her what associations she had with teddy bears. She said: "None. I think I had one as a kid, but I don't remember being that attached to it." So I invited her to imagine she was a preverbal infant and to explore that teddy bear as if she were seeing it for the first time.

Maralies had a good sense of drama. She rubbed the teddy bear all over her body, even lifting her shirt to feel it on her belly. She put one paw in her mouth and sucked on it. She gazed into the teddy bear's eyes. She put it over her nose and inhaled deeply; she hugged it and made baby sounds, cooing and squealing with delight.

After about ten minutes, she said: "I'm not sure what I'm doing here, and this is extremely weird, but I felt my gut unclenching and the pain in my intestines went from six to three on the pain scale."

We retested her energy systems and now they were all even stronger. We tried the same thing with a few other objects sitting around my office: a water glass, a pen, a toy porcupine. With each experiment, doing some basic sensorimotor exploration caused the energies to strengthen and her gut to feel better. After about twenty minutes, her gut was no longer hurting her.

Energetic responses to the world are often passed down from generation to generation, which is one reason addictions, illnesses, and psychological problems seem to run in families. Part of what was happening for

Maralies was that a learned level of danger and stress (probably from her grandmother Elsa) was built into whatever other understandings she had gained of the world. Because it was built in at a preverbal, unarticulated level, it was nearly invisible to her.

Although she could explain that her grandmother had been a terrified perfectionist, and her mother was a get-ahead perfectionist, she never realized that her own relationship to the world included those same stresses, coded into everything she did. The focus on getting ahead that was pure survival for her grandmother, and that was emotional survival for her mother, translated for Maralies as a need to push through and quickly master experiences, rather than relaxing to just live them. She had racked up all kinds of accomplishments but did not give herself permission to just be with things and let go of expectations.

That became her self-care task for a while. To let herself have sensorimotor time. To put aside the notion that she needed to heal her gut and immune system, and instead to just listen to her gut reactions as she directly encountered the world around her. She needed to provide safe explorations with no ulterior motive or goal: just experience for the sake of experience. She decided to do this both as an imaginary infant in the privacy of her home and as an attitude to take into her everyday life as best she could.

Within a month, Maralies was able to report that her Crohn's was in remission and her lupus-like symptoms had not flared. With the support of some additional energy medicine tools to keep her feeling safe, she reported after a year that the Crohn's was gone, as was the lupus.

Not all disconnects from direct experience come from our early years. Even if your sensorimotor phase was joyous and supported, it is useful to ask yourself how directly and fully you are able to experience your life now. As we grow from infant to young child to student to adult, we often end up transferring gratification from the thing itself to a symbol. So instead of feeling satisfaction while learning at school, we anticipate and experience the joy of getting a good grade and symbolic approval from parents and teachers. Instead of feeling deep pleasure and satisfaction with each bite of a good meal, we are busy posting photos of it on Instagram or counting calories to assure ourselves eating it is really on our diet plan. Instead of enjoying a hug and cuddle, we sometimes go through the motions while calculating whether this means our partner has gotten over the fight we had yesterday.

The stress of being cut off from direct encounter can mess up your body's energy communications. It can cause your body to oversignal needs or cause you to miss signals of *enough*. So it is useful to drop back into that pure sense of direct encounter from time to time throughout the day. Tune in to things you encounter with all your senses. Explore the *now* in intimate detail. It can nourish and renew you at a baseline level. This is a crucial building block in how you construct wellness and use the language of energy.

TOTAL IMMERSION

Learning language involves both comprehension and expression.

Young children are totally immersed in a world of language that is spoken to them and surrounds them. They comprehend far more than they are taught directly, learning to distinguish specifics from the whole field of language and communication they are exposed to.

They learn to express themselves by constructing language from the ground up: first by learning to produce sounds, then holophrases (single words that communicate a whole concept), then basic two-word sentences, then telegraphic sentences, then joined sentences that link specifics, then overgeneralizations, and on and on.

In learning the language of energy, it is useful to recognize that you are also going through a similar two-pronged process. Your task is to build both *comprehension*, deepening your ability to perceive subtle energies in the fields that surround you, and *expression*, developing your ability to communicate using subtle energies.

Too often people learning energy healing (either for self-help or to work with others) just study methods and techniques. They put tools in their tool kits and miss the essentials of both developing their subtle perceptions *and* constructing an individualized ability to communicate with energies. It is like memorizing phrases rather than learning to converse.

Fortunately, learning to perceive and speak energy is not difficult. You have already gained fluency in at least one language, so your mind is familiar with the process. And your body already communicates with itself using energy:

- Your mind-body-spirit conducts ongoing consultations that are energetic in nature.
- You communicate energetically with people around you, both consciously and below your awareness.
- You move through various energetic fields or atmospheres that are palpable as you encounter them during your day.

Learning (or remembering) the language of energy is a matter of tuning in, awakening to the constant energetic expressions and exchanges, and letting your instinctive abilities help you to gain skill in active expression.

Your body is designed to perceive energies using all your senses and receptive faculties (which I discuss in chapter 3):

- Seeing, either with your mind's eye or physical eye
- Hearing, either literally or in your imagination
- Smell
- Taste
- Touch, feeling, and physical sensation
- Direct knowing
- Intuitive hits
- Animal instinct
- Attention, or being drawn to notice something
- Energy shifts, or recognizing changes in pattern or affect

Further, you can communicate with your body's energies using the following energy vocabulary (which I explore in chapters 4 through 6):

- Touch
- Gesture
- Imagery, symbols, visualization

- Light and color
- Sound
- Rhythm
- Movement
- Breath
- Shapes
- Scent
- Taste
- Intention that helps guide behaviors of subtle energies
- Field energies, including environmental placement and nature

• • • PLAY WITH IT • • •

Find a place in your body that is uncomfortable or catching your attention in this moment. Notice how you tune in to it: Are you feeling your way in? Scanning your body with your mind? Getting a mental image? Perhaps your mind just went directly to the place, or you thought, *My left knee.* Each of us perceives in unique ways, so it is useful to get to know your go-to style of perceiving.

As you tune in to the place in your body, what sensations is it communicating to you? You might feel pain, tightness, heat, or vibration. You might see a color, hear sounds, or smell something. Open your mind to whatever and however that place in your body is communicating. Some people get images or even messages as that part of the body speaks to them.

Now, review the above list of ways you can communicate with subtle energies. Choose one to experiment with.

Example: When I do this, my attention is called to my left knee because it feels tight and sore; my eyes are pulled there, too. Looking over the list of communication tools, I feel drawn to "rhythm." So, I listen to my inner being for a moment to see if a rhythm wants to emerge, and the rhythm I hear or feel drawn to is the *lub-dub* rhythm of the heart.

I tap using this *lub-dub* rhythm all around the knee. Because it is a heart rhythm, I place my other hand on my heart, intensifying the linkage between my heart *lub-dub* and the *lub-dub* I am tapping on my knee. I experiment: Does it feel better when I tap with my fingertips or my palms? Do I want light taps or sharper staccato ones? Or would I rather just hold my knee while playing a strong rhythmic beat on the table next to me?

When you play with this, at a certain point in your experimentation, you will feel done or else drawn to another tool. Keep tuning in to the body part to see how it is feeling and what it wants. The goal is not necessarily to *fix* the problem but to *respond* to it, to open to what your body is communicating and dialogue lovingly with it using the language of energy.

• • • • • •

PRACTICE TIPS

The language of energy is not a foreign language, though it might seem that way at first, if you are used to thinking about your body in chemical, biological terms. Since it is our first language, learning it is a combination of awakening to what you already do to communicate with yourself energetically and of building on that situationally, the way an infant learns language.

- Track all the ways your body communicates with you throughout a twenty-four-hour period. Does it signal with aches or pains? Does it send sensations of hunger or fatigue, aversion or attraction? Do you feel like it pulls the plug or puts you into overdrive to get your conscious attention? Does it fidget or tighten muscles? Does it stumble, drop things, shift your mood, play movies in your head? Like getting acquainted with an infant, explore how your physical self signals desires and needs.
- When stress shows up in your mind or body, take a few minutes to respond with direct energetic communication: tapping, stroking, crooning, or bathing in a soothing color,

sound, shape, gesture, or smell. What consolation can you bring it, as you would a screaming infant?

- Several times a day, drop into a sensorimotor experience of the world. Tune in to see, feel, hear, smell, and taste what is unfolding in your now. Turn off thoughts and just focus on direct encounter.

- Spend a few moments describing your parents, grandparents (and even great-grandparents, if you can). What descriptors best fit each of them and their energy? Was Grandma tense and controlling? Was Grandpa expansive and invasive? How do those energetic qualities play out in or influence you?

- Make a list of what gratifies you. Then sort the items into three groups: (1) objects, people, or actions that gratify you through direct experience; (2) ideas that gratify you; and (3) gratification that comes as a result of achieving a goal or aspiration. Notice where most of your gratification comes from. Make an effort to find more moments of direct gratification throughout your day: Taste your food, sink into the comfort of a nap, play with your dog or child with undivided attention. Notice what happens to your sense of connection and gratification when you are multitasking or delaying gratification to power through the moment.

Chapter Three

SENSING SUBTLE ENERGIES

My clients have been all over the map with how they perceive energies. I've worked with confirmed skeptics who could feel into their subtle energies with beautiful precision, and I've worked with fervent believers who were pretty much tone-deaf to their own inner communications. But with practice, and perhaps some guidance on how to proceed, almost everyone can develop a working ability to perceive energies.

The jumping-off place to learn to perceive subtle energies is to understand that you are already doing it! Your body reacts to danger before your conscious mind has parsed the situation and decided it is dangerous. Your ears pick up vibration and tone of voice and interpret it as *attitude* when someone is speaking. You know, when someone says, "That's sick," whether they mean something is unhealthy or extremely positive (using slang). You can usually tell when someone's touch is friendly or controlling, reassuring or threatening.

Sensing subtle energies has often been linked to being psychic. But it is more akin to our everyday perceptions. If I can perceive that a washcloth is wet, and easily distinguish between that and a dry one, why wouldn't

I be able to transfer that skill and recognize water element in someone's being (which I explain in chapter 9) and distinguish dampness or dryness as qualities of someone's energies?

• • • PLAY WITH IT • • •

Think of five people you know well. Using your instincts and overall impressions, rank them on a range from dry to wet. Who is the driest of the five? Then list the next driest, the one in the middle range, and the two who are most wet.

Try this ranking with other qualities. Among those five people, who is the most contracted and who is more relaxed? Who is the most expansive? Is the most expansive person also the biggest in physical size? Ranking energies and qualities is not based on physical traits alone, but on our sense of someone's spirit, personality, or energy style.

Who is the most energetic, and how do you rank the five people on a scale from most energetic to the least energetic? You may or may not know why you rank each person the way you do. Are you using active, explicit criteria or pure instinct? Both are valid.

Whenever you notice a trait in someone, explore it in others. Someone may say to you, "Annette lives a very small life." What does that feel like? Who do you know who lives a bigger life? What do you base that sense on?

We often mix our subjective and objective observations. We mix our perceptions of energies with assessments of behaviors (which are energetic expressions), and we base our perceptions on language as well. It is not cheating to mix and match these.

For example, when I think of a certain friend, the word that comes to mind is *steadfast*. How would I rank my other friends and acquaintances on that scale of steadfast to unreliable (which describes a certain quality of energy)? When I think about those other friends who are not quite as steadfast, what words characterize their energies most accurately?

• • • • • •

EXPLORING SUBTLE ENERGIES: YOUR SENSES

To begin exploring subtle energies more consciously, tune in to your body to sense what is going on energetically. You can use the perceptions of your everyday senses as an entry point: seeing, hearing, smelling, tasting, and feeling. You may perceive a literal, physical sensation, such as, say, a sudden sensation of cold that makes you shiver, or your perception may be more internal: seeing in your mind's eye, hearing a sound or voice in your head, feeling a sensation you can recognize but that is not quite physical, tasting something in your mouth or smelling something that you know is not literally there.

You may already have a pretty nuanced ability to perceive using your senses and inner senses. For example, can you see something yellow and recognize whether it is sunshine yellow or sickly yellow? Can you hear a tune in your head and recognize the mood of it? No matter what your starting point, the more you tune in to your perceptions and investigate them, the more nuance you will come to recognize.

Seeing

I am not particularly visual in my *seeing*. I know what the color is in my mind, but I don't usually visualize it strongly. My artist friends often see color on an inner canvas, and for them it rarely limits itself to just color: It takes on form, patterns, and dimension.

However, whether a sense is strong or weak for you, consider the quality of it. When you see a color, what do you see about it? Is it bright or dark? Is it still or moving? And if it is moving, how is it moving? Is it a healthy form of that color or one that your mind finds unsettling in some way? Ask similar questions as you experiment with each sense.

• • • PLAY WITH IT • • •

Find a place in your body that wants to talk to you. Just let your hand hover over your body until it lands on a location. It is useful to turn off your logical mind for this activity. Let instinct guide you. For some people who process things primarily through their intellect, that can be nearly impossible. If so, include your logical brain in the game. Shut your eyes and ask your brain: *Where does my hand want to land?*

With your hand on that place (which helps your perceptions focus into the energies there), *look* to see what color you perceive. For most people, it works best to shut your eyes and use your inner vision. If you experiment doing this with your eyes open, you may find a color entering your field of vision that is not the color of your clothing. Play with it. Do you see or sense a color?

Note that some people can't activate their other senses while touching an area because their kinesthetic sense is so strong. If that is true for you, just touch the area briefly, then explore using your inner vision to tune in. Once you sense a color, evaluate and explore all of its qualities.

Example: When I do this, my hand wants to go to my right ear and cover it. I do not have pain there. In fact, it feels much clearer than my left ear. But I shut my eyes and tune in where my hand lands and see a dark gray color, almost the absence of color. The color is still, like before the dawn. I ask what it wants. At first, it is just very still and gray. Nothing moves. I wait to see if what it wants is to just be in a gray suspended state. For a minute or two, it hovers in that gray. Then, I see a yellow light entering. It is full sunlight yellow filtering into the field of gray and dappling it. Then the picture shifts to green foliage with yellow sunlight filtering through. I find it soothing and peaceful. And I realize, as I sit cupping my right ear, that a sadness in my heart due to the recent death of my cat is shifting to a quiet, peaceful feeling. Like hanging out in a green bower, protected from direct sun, but watching it play all around me.

I don't know what my right ear has to do with my heart, or my cat, but allowing my hands and subtle energies to guide a process of transformation helps me move a piece of grief and transform it into a different energetic state. I know that the next time I feel the sadness, I can imagine myself once again in the green bower to find comfort, or I can tune in to the sadness once again and ask for further guidance.

• • • • • •

Sensations Are Communications

Notice that I ask, *What does this color want or need?* Sometimes I ask, *What does it want to become?* The color I perceive represents a subtle energy that's communicating with me.

I prefer these questions, rather than asking, *What do I want the color to become?* I can ask how the color makes me feel, or what I register as its meaning, but too often my brain leaps in with thoughts about what I think I want, and these desires aren't necessarily in keeping with my soul's or body's purpose. My mind might think, *It needs to be bright yellow, like sunshine.* But the color may want to dull its shade to moon yellow in accordance with some communication I don't yet understand.

You may also notice I am not limiting this activity to pure perception. Even if you are doing an exercise focused on a particular sense, it is still a moment of tuning in to a subtle energy. Remember, these are the energies that make up your web of meaning. Therefore, it is a moment of communion with meaning — the doorway to communication. So when I see an energy in my body and ask what it wants or needs, I am responding to it *as a communication*, as an expression of a truth in the moment, and not treating it as static. If it wants or needs me to just witness it, I will sense that. Or it won't shift when I invite it to shift. Then I can dig deeper into what I am seeing: *Okay, that's the color. What else can I notice about it?*

Hearing

You can similarly use your *hearing* to tune in and listen to an area of your body. You might be picking up sounds, hearing a song that expresses what the energies are doing, perceiving a rhythm, or even hearing words or a voice that can guide you. Use whatever vocabulary you have relating to sound to help you pick up and recognize the communications of your subtle energies.

One great aspect of using hearing is that often your subtle energies will talk to you. But like any dialogue, you get more information if you ask open-ended questions rather than yes/no questions, and let it unfold as dialogue rather than looking for immediate right answers. An open-ended question asks, for example, "Can you give me insight into [fill in the blank]?" I like to joke that you wouldn't hike up a mountain to see a wise guru in a cave, only to say, "In one word, tell me the meaning of life," or, "I'd like you to explain the meaning of life to me, so I'm going to ask you some yes/no questions, and you can tell me if I'm right."

If open-ended questions don't yield insight, you can guide the dialogue a bit by asking questions about what you're hearing that might expand your understanding: *Is your volume what it needs to be? Is the balance of sound okay here? Is there movement or rhythm, and is the rhythm you're hearing the one that is most needed here? Are you pulsing or vibrating the way you want to?*

Like with perceiving colors, you are not looking to define what is wrong. You are trying to perceive what *is* (and what is becoming, since all energy moves), with as much detail as you can supply, using your everyday skills and senses. Focus on understanding what's being communicated, by asking: *Is there something you need? Can I do something for you? Is there something you need me to know?*

• • • PLAY WITH IT • • •

Let your hand move to a part of your body that seems to want to communicate with you. Use either your literal ears or your inner sense of hearing (like you can hear the voice of a beloved friend in your mind) to tune in. Is there a tone or note or even song associated with the area? Are there words that come to mind? Is it noise or sound or music? Is it resonant, like a tone, or rhythmic, like a drumbeat, or both?

Example: My hand goes straight to my gut, where my small intestine is ringed by my large intestine. I listen in and hear a kind of occasional slow release: *blip…blip…blip….* As I keep listening, I hear this chorus singing in the background, kind of like workers singing to keep their energies steady as they work. I listen to the music, but can't quite make out the words or tune. Does it need something from me? I hear the word *appreciation*, and the thought occurs to me that I spend a lot of time worrying about my gut, but in fact it is working away down there, doing its job. So I feel a moment of gratitude and notice a sudden release of tension throughout my torso. Could it be I haven't been trusting those blipping workers to do their jobs?

The rhythm of the blips interests me. It's like a very slow march. I experiment with tapping that rhythm on my trunk, arms, and legs. It feels good. I'm not sure what I am doing, but I feel like my body has just shown me something about the rhythm of my digestive system: It is slower and more deliberate than my mind, which tends to race. I find that tapping my foot in that rhythm also relaxes me, both physically and mentally.

• • • • • • •

Smell and Taste

Smell and *taste* follow similar patterns. I have had clients who could smell energies as I worked with them. While I cleared a meridian related to earth energy, they said: "I smell soil" (or manure, loam, or dry dust). I've also had clients who complained of certain tastes in their mouths that turned out to reveal which element was out of balance (based on the five elements of Chinese medicine).

Certain sayings reflect how we use taste and smell to perceive energies: "That experience left a bad taste in my mouth." "This situation doesn't smell right." As someone who has always loved to eat, I have a varied palate that I can use in perceiving subtle energies this way.

• • • PLAY WITH IT • • •

Tune in to your body and let your hand move to a place that wants to communicate. Now use your senses of taste and smell to give you information. Is the place you are touching spicy or bland? What kind of flavor is it (salty, sweet, sour, bitter, hot)? What is the aroma of the energy? How nourishing is it? Like testing a good wine, you can *taste and smell* energies and recognize component parts. You might think: *The energy I'm picking up here tastes smooth and bitter, and I am picking up a slight scent of cinnamon.* As with vision and sound, you can ask what spices or flavors or scents might be of service to the energies in question. Or maybe what is needed is something that will clear the air or clear the palate!

Imagine you are a sniffer dog like the ones checking for contraband at the airport. Send your sense of smell into each part of your body to sniff out energetic issues. Then using whatever information comes to you, play with your responses. You might want to set up a fan to clear out a fuggy smell. You might look to see if something is rotting (like forgotten leftovers in the back of the refrigerator). Can you use your hands to energetically pull out the container and wash away the stink? Do you need to open windows to let in a breeze?

• • • • • •

Scents Make Sense

Kay was sensitive to scents, particularly perfumes and chemical scents. Riding in an elevator with people wearing perfume could leave her with a terrible headache and shortness of breath. New carpets left her dizzy and disoriented. The problem was causing her to avoid situations where she might be exposed to perfumes, such as going to the theater. She confessed that at night, as she was trying to go to sleep, she would be overwhelmed by the smell of feces, even though she had just showered and had clean sheets.

This did not surprise me. In Chinese medicine the sense of smell is governed by metal element, which embraces both large intestine and lung energies. She was smelling her own imbalance. We tried several methods to rebalance her metal element. And as energy shifted, I noticed Kay was giving commentary on smells: "I'm smelling a sharp, sour smell....Now I smell something sweet." I realized that Kay had a supersensitive gift for smell, and so when our efforts to rebalance her metal element wouldn't hold, we decided to try a different approach: balancing it from the inside by letting it guide her.

I invited Kay to tune in to parts of her body and tell me what smell came to her. That was easy for her. I invited her to ask the smell what was needed or wanted. She would find herself transported in her mind to another environment with a different odor. After a few minutes of using this antidote smell, the original smell would dissipate. It was fascinating for me to see that the meridian energies governing the original smell would also shift.

Using her nose to guide her explorations became Kay's self-care tool. She discovered that if she breathed in the smell of her own wrist, she was able to be around other scents without getting knocked off-balance. It was a clever way to bring herself home to her own perceptions. Over time, she was able to teach her immune system to stop overreacting to scents by using her gift more consciously and more often. The more she developed her gift, the less oversensitive she became to unwanted inputs. She got better at tuning out unnecessary scent information the way our ears and brain can learn to tune out sounds that aren't relevant to us. She also learned to see her sense of smell as the gift it was and stop beating herself up for her vulnerability.

When I last saw her, Kay had found a balance between participating in events she wanted to attend, such as theater; asking people not to wear scents when that was possible; and using energy medicine exercises and her own wrist antidote to bring herself back in balance when she was unexpectedly hit by unavoidable scents.

Energy dialogue often flourishes if we can play with the inputs and use our imagination, hands, and symbolic movements to respond to what we are discovering.

You can use both taste and smell descriptors in a kind of metaphoric sense, and you might literally taste or smell the energies you are tuning in to. Because we eat several times a day, these two senses are highly developed in most people, and yet we don't use them enough to understand what we are picking up about someone's energies. Is the person delicious or bland? What flavor or scent do you associate in your mind with that person?

Touch, Feeling, and Physical Sensation

Feeling, physical and emotional sensation, is especially useful in perceiving energies. Your skin is considered the largest sense organ of the body. (I actually see the aura as a sense organ, which is larger, but we can recognize both are big sense organs!) Like with the other senses, you can perceive with your skin directly or feel sensations with your inner sense of feeling. Think of a time when you felt an inner burn, even though your skin wasn't registering heat. It is no accident that we frequently ask others how they are feeling. The word refers to both the sensations of the body and to the emotions. Feelings reflect your understanding of energies and your relationship to your inner landscape.

The ability to process information via sensation is called *kinesthetic*. You can use your kinesthetic sense in several ways:

- You can use your hands to *scan* someone else's body and energies, picking up information via these amazing two-way communication devices.
- You can tune in to your own body to read sensations that are reflections of what someone else is feeling. (I am quite kinesthetic, so I often have to stop and figure out whether the pain I am feeling is mine or an echo of someone else's pain registering in my kinesthetic receivers.)
- You can feel your way into someone else's subtle energies intuitively and interpret what you are picking up via your ability to interpret feelings and sensations. In this latter case, it is most likely you are using your aura or energy field as a sense organ because our auras intermingle with those of other people, and the influence of their subtle energies touching ours can give us a lot of information.
- You can use your ability to feel (or any of your sense organs, for that matter) via a form of resonance, where your senses pick up the energetic vibration of someone else's subtle energies at a distance and briefly register those sensations in your own body. This is often used in distance healing work.

Many people are uncomfortable with openly acknowledging sensations. We medicate our bodies at the first sign of pain; we shy away from visibly feeling pleasurable sensations in public. Have you ever felt embarrassed because someone is saying "Oooooooh" out loud in public, in response to a friend's shoulder rub or a delicious flavor? We fall down and immediately assure everyone who rushes to help that we are fine, before we have even investigated what is hurting. Many of us often ignore symptoms that might guide us back to health because we don't want to admit we are not feeling right.

• • • PLAY WITH IT • • •

To explore feeling, imagine you have sensors on your hands: in your palms, in your fingertips, and even in your skin. You can scan someone's energy field, working just half an inch or so off the skin, to get information about their energy.

Scan yourself with your hands. Are you feeling heat or cool, stillness or movement, rhythmic or arrhythmic patterns, bumpy or smooth, dense or diffuse, and so on? Like the Halloween game where someone is blindfolded and plunges their hands into bowls of stuff like cold spaghetti, olives, and Jell-O, you can strive to identify what you are feeling.

With feeling and feelings, the goal is to gather information about the energy, and as described with the other senses, dialogue with it. We can dialogue not only by asking questions with our minds, but also by letting our hands do the talking. Often if you let your hands just go, they will naturally bring healing energy in, try to untangle knots, get blocked energy moving, separate energies that are glommed together, and otherwise bring relief.

• • • • • •

EXPLORING SUBTLE ENERGIES:
DIRECT KNOWING AND INTUITIVE HITS

Our abilities to sense and perceive energies go beyond the five senses acknowledged in Western culture. The mind itself is a sense organ that receives information via direct knowing and thoughts. This may involve telepathy, where someone sends you a thought or image and your mind receives it, or it might involve the ability of your Talking Self to travel to other dimensions of consciousness and gather information.

I have known healers who are able to use their dreams (or trance journeying) to gather all kinds of information about a health condition for themselves or a loved one. Some might argue that this is the brain itself or the subconscious working in the background, but I suspect it is a sixth sense that is part of the energetic exchange built into our Talking Self dimension.

We can imagine our way into someone's body (with their permission) and get information about it. We can open to our intuition, which might just be another name for the whole array of receptors we possess, and let symbolic hits inform our understanding.

These intuitive hits often come as one word, one image, or one sensation.

Note: It is important to always get explicit permission from a person before scanning them energetically. You wouldn't pull down someone's pants to check out their underwear, so please give someone's energies the same courtesy. Asking their spirit for permission is usually not adequate. If you want to practice these skills, it is best to practice on yourself or willing friends and family members who clearly give you permission to do so.

• • • PLAY WITH IT • • •

As before, tune in to an area of your body. Open your mind to whatever thought, word, image, or sensation comes to you. You are asking for insight, not necessarily what you should do or what is wrong. The trick with opening to intuition is to let information in without judging it, then afterward, unpack the meaning or try to understand what light it might shed. Often there is a time lapse, so it's good to keep a notebook with intuitive hits and give them time to unfold in your conscious mind.

Example: When I tune in to my stomach area, I get an immediate image of something exploding in a starburst pattern, like a firework. It is a positive explosion, not a problem. This hit speaks to me right away on one level: It's a need to give out rather than take in. It's a need to celebrate and sparkle and share and send my energies in many directions. I will sit with this intuitive hit for a while and check back in occasionally to see if the image shifts or if it is acting as a guiding star over a period of time. In the short term, I will spend some time freewriting, just to generate ideas, because it feels like the stomach area of my web of meaning is asking me to express myself in many directions — like distributing nutrients out to my whole field rather than clutching everything in a tight fist at the solar plexus. I've been getting the closed fist message for that area over and over recently.

• • • • • •

Your Aura as a Sense Organ

I have observed that the aura itself, being a field of meaning that moves, vibrates, and resonates, can register energies that are not part of its own circulating patterns. Just as if you are singing a song and hear a different tune, you can usually tell that the other tune is not part of your song. You can hear two different songs at once. By the same token, the consciousness that manages your energy field can perceive what is you and what is not you, differentiate the two, and hear both realities.

You have probably experienced this. Imagine you are in a great mood. You are walking down the street and pass someone you barely notice visually. Suddenly you feel a chill, as if the sun has gone behind the clouds. You look up and the sky is clear. You check in with yourself and your own energies are still humming. But you are also feeling the chill you just passed. Most likely someone with disturbed or frozen energies just passed you, and your aura briefly resonated with that second energy state, while holding on to the truth of your original tune.

To help your aura hold its own, see "Reinforcing the Smart Filter of the Aura" (page 205).

EXPLORING SUBTLE ENERGIES: INSTINCTS, ATTENTION, AND ENERGY SHIFTS

Your Earth Elemental Self has a built-in guidance system that helps you maintain physicality. It also has guidance from your Talking Self (the conscious mind) and Wiser Self. Sometimes these three sources of guidance differ and create conflicts. That's easy enough to see. Your body is feeling tired and pulling you to take a nap. Talking Self is telling you to drink coffee so you can get another hour of work in. And Wiser Self may be pulling you into a reverie where you can already picture yourself on vacation, swinging in a hammock next to a tropical beach.

Your inner guidance system often speaks by activating your animal instincts, drawing your attention to something, or flagging an energy shift in pattern or affect. You might notice you are hearing or feeling a sudden change in your environment. You might feel a shift in your mood, or in your perceptions about what is happening around you. You might feel an instinctive urge to withdraw or notice a sudden craving. We are designed to get ongoing feedback and guidance about what is going on with the circulation of our subtle energies and in the creation of our web of meaning.

However, our physical instincts get drowned out in a culture where light and dark no longer track the movements of the sun, and where patterns of activity and rest don't correlate to direct survival needs. How is your body to interpret a life-or-death battle you are watching on Netflix at the end of a long workday? What are you asking of it chemically? It doesn't easily differentiate the energy of imagined reality from the energy of physical reality because it is programmed to embody the agendas of all three selves.

In light of this, self-healing often requires us to learn to attune more directly to our instinct, to our creature nature. Like returning to a sensorimotor activity to recharge in direct experience, turning off the Talking Self agendas and letting yourself be a creature, aligning your rhythms with very physical events, can be deeply healing. Have you ever felt yourself getting sick and found that some very physical, mindless task, like raking leaves, actually made you feel better? Your physical task resets your body's communications, which in turn calms the immune system that is gearing up to force you to pay attention and take some downtime.

I had a meditation teacher, Ruth Denison, who often helped mentally ill people recover without medications by setting them very physical tasks.[2] She would say: "Sweep the porch. Know you are holding the broom. Know you are moving the broom. Feel the broom move the dirt along the floorboard. Feel the end of the movement as you shift, lift the broom, start again." This is a form of mindfulness practice that allows the Earth Elemental Self to reset your instincts and to work in harmony with Talking Self, calming your mind and reorganizing patterns that were spinning you out of touch with this dimension of reality.

As you learn to tune in to your instincts, you can assess how often you support your creature self and how often you contravene it. If you watch a dog or cat, they seem to have such clear guidance: *Now it is time to nap. Now it is time to check out the food bowl. Now it is time to lick and clean my fur. Now it is time to get a cuddle. Now it is time to play with the toy.* The perpetual now is healing to the creature self, which in turn houses your mind and spirit. In the now, you can generally hear simple, clear guidance.

• • • PLAY WITH IT • • •

Place one hand on your heart and one hand on your solar plexus. Turn off your thinking brain for a moment and ask your body what it needs *now*. If you tune in, your instrument can show you what it needs now, often in clear pictures or in short suggestions: rest, snack, lie down, stretch, yawn, move, breathe, sleep, shut eyes, go to the bathroom, hug someone. It can guide you, moment by moment, into balance.

Example: I feel tired from not sleeping well the night before, and my mind suggests: *green tea*. I tune in to my body for guidance and expect her to signal the obvious: nap. But she surprises me: She wants me to lie down and do what I call "three-five breathing." This is breathing in on a count of three and out on a count of five. As I do this, I feel my body shifting into four-eight breathing, and within about five minutes I feel renewed, as though I have had a nap.

• • • • • •

Using the breath is often a great way to reset the inner guidance system. Going into nature in a relaxed way can also accomplish this: lean against a tree, walk barefoot in the sand or grass, sit and contemplate the sky or a vista, walk slowly through a park. Or pull yourself into the now by acting like your dog or cat and inhabiting each moment for a time: *Now it is time to stretch my arms and legs and back. Now it is time to look out the window. Now it is time to notice I am breathing. Now it is time to step outside into the sun. Now it is time to revel in mindless joy.*

Your Guidance System Is Rooted in Instinct

Our instincts work through attraction and aversion. Our attention is drawn to something — we are meant to pay attention. Our instincts tell us to move away from something — we are meant to avoid it. When the instincts are working correctly, we can trust what we crave and resist.

But when your energies are out of balance, your instincts go out of balance as well: You crave things you don't need and resist things you do. If the situation is chronic enough, the whole guidance system can turn on itself, just as a rabbit caught in a trap will chew off its own foot. This is the root of autoimmune illness: When the inner guidance system can't be heard, the immune system can turn and start to attack the body it is meant to protect.

Many of the energy medicine exercises offered throughout this book help to rebalance your basic energy systems, so you can perceive your inner guidance and instincts again. See in particular: "Porcupine Reset" (page 201), "Yin Hearts" (page 198), "Reinforcing the Smart Filter of the Aura" (page 205), "Seven Spirals" (page 225), "Earth Dock–Sky Dock" (page 212), and "Suit Reboot" (page 230).

SELF-HEALING VIA ENERGY DIALOGUE

The mantra of self-healing via energy dialogue is: *Tune in. Listen. Perceive what the energies are doing or asking for. Respond appropriately.*

This is such a different approach than going from practitioner to practitioner trying to find out what is wrong, trying to find the magic bullet (or pill) that will stop the skewed communications of a body screaming to be heard. The body calls attention to what needs to be heard, witnessed, supported, and perhaps responded to in loving dialogue. That transaction happens repeatedly, not just in a morning routine of exercises or in an afternoon hands-on treatment.

As you tune in regularly, you will start to notice patterns. For instance, you may notice you often lose your focus at 10 AM, or that your jaw gets tight when you meet with people who are high energy. One key way that subtle energies communicate is to signal shifts: in patterns, in energy behaviors, in your mood. We aren't meant to track all the movement of all our energies at all times. Just as we scan a visual landscape and focus on a few specifics, rather than trying to see every detail in front of us, our consciousness is designed to signal significant shifts.

Therefore, perceiving subtle energies is often most productive when you invite your hands and your senses to show you the way. It is also a highly productive way to engage in energy dialogue. When a mood shifts, when we feel energies rise, fall, or change their rhythm, those are all times to tune in to hear what is being signaled and what the inner-guidance system is requesting.

All chronic illness (and much acute illness) is due to miscommunication, or *missed communion,* so the solutions to our health challenges often rest in our ability to find communion with the energies that we are made of: the miraculous creation of self happening endlessly within us. There is a lot of power in being the witness, in showing up.

While the language of energy has more complex tools and techniques, if your goal is to take healing into your own hands, it can be a powerful baseline practice to tap into the simple and direct guidance system built into your creature self and allow the wisdom in it to guide you forward.

PRACTICE TIPS

- If you tune in and don't see, hear, smell, taste, feel, or know anything, just visit and dwell in the space for a while. Sometimes it's enough to just show up; awareness comes later.
- If you feel blocked in your ability to tune in, try "Clear Fear, Ease Ego, Welcome Wiser Self" (page 148).
- If you get images or colors and don't know what they mean, just note them down in a journal and keep tuning in over time. Your infant self didn't understand spoken language at

first, either — but over time your comprehension grew, and the same will happen with this language, too!

- If you feel worried about what you see (say, a scene of devastation), understand you are in the metaphoric or symbolic realm. Images are a representation of the energies as they are and as they are becoming. Keep asking what is needed to move you toward wholeness. This style of dialogue is *not* prediction.

- The language of the guiding self is individual. If you try to look up the symbols or colors in a book, that is turning to outside authority. Chances are your Earth Elemental Self has not read that book and isn't using the symbols or colors the way the book's author describes!

- The goal of this work is not to fix your energies but to encounter them and have a heartfelt, loving, supportive dialogue. If you are using these techniques to dig out faults and weaknesses, it will only discourage your Earth Elemental Self from trusting you.

- Remember: Sickness is a falling away from wellness. Keep asking for insights into what wellness feels and looks like, which I discuss in more detail later.

Chapter Four

SPEAK YOUR BODY'S LANGUAGE

First Words

You already communicate with energies and practice energy medicine instinctively. When you put your hands on the sides of your face to comfort yourself, you are talking to two or three different energy streams (meridians) and reaching deeper to one of the flows that feeds them called Penetrating Flow. When you are alarmed and put your hand to your forehead, you are covering and activating points that help calm emotions. When you are winded and bend over with your hands on your knees, back flat, you are grounding your energy, calming your nervous system, and opening up the energy stream that sends resources to the brain, as well as letting gravity support your lungs. But however much you speak energy instinctively, healing with energy is more effective if you learn to use it more consciously.

Back in the 1970s a psychologist wanted to figure out how boys in their early teens could learn to express a greater range of emotions. She was curious whether the boys had difficulty *feeling* emotions or whether, in fact, they just lacked the vocabulary or skill to express them. She gave them a list of words that expressed a whole diverse universe of emotions. What she discovered was that once they had the words, they were able to talk about their feelings and affirm that they did in fact feel. They felt a lot.

Without a baseline vocabulary for the language of energy, we become like those young teenage boys: unable to participate with breadth and depth in our own energetic experiences.

Developmental psychologists say children learn to speak (and think) by *constructing their language,* incorporating new concepts by scaffolding onto what already exists. Just as an infant constructs language from simple words up, you can learn the language of energy best by starting with basic vocabulary and playing with those basics until you can create your own meaningful usage. As an adult, you will learn self-healing more deeply if you also construct your own ways to communicate with your subtle energies and scaffold this language onto your own unique experiential base.

THE RIGHT TOOL FOR THE JOB

Myra worked for a government agency in a high-stress position. In her limited spare time, she took care of her aging mother. The stress was starting to erode her health. She suffered from insomnia and had anxiety attacks when she tried to relax. She had developed a strange skin disorder and noticed her hair was thinning at a rate greater than normal.

When we assessed her energies, it seemed like she could only hold strong by staying on high alert. When she took a deep breath and exhaled, the relaxation actually made her energies go into reactivity. That is not an uncommon pattern. Migraine sufferers tend to get migraines on their days off, holding it together during the work week. Myra was a woman with a strong will, and as long as she was doing things for others, she found she could hold it together, apart from the signs of erosion her body was expressing.

Myra could not handle a whole list of self-care exercises — she barely had time to accomplish what she was already doing, and she was unwilling to take anything off her plate. So we discussed the possibility of finding ways to walk through her day with a different energy. Instead of holding it together by keeping herself tightly strung, what if she could strengthen her core to make everything feel easier?

I taught Myra about her core note. This is the vibration at which each person's deepest energy system, their grid, resonates. It is unique for each person. The "Core Note" exercise (page 96) appealed to Myra because she could sing or hum at work even while doing other things.

We experimented and found that singing her core note overrode the energetic collapse that was happening when she relaxed. Our plan was to have her try singing her core note each time she felt she was white-knuckling her day. Then we would reconvene in a week or two and assess what else could serve.

We kept that first appointment simple, focused on hearing what her system wanted and needed *now*.

Myra didn't come back for six months. When she showed up again, I asked if she was okay with the earlier appointment. She laughed! "It was great," she said. "That core note did the trick, so I didn't need any other tools. I sing it every day whenever I feel like it, and for some reason, it makes my job feel much easier. And my skin cleared up, my hair stopped falling out, and the anxiety attacks and insomnia stopped."

She was back now for another tool because her mother had declined and was in hospice, and she was getting overwhelmed. This time around, she was open to rethinking what was on her plate; she could imagine new options.

Self-healing is not always so simple. But often, if you find the right tool for the moment, you have a precious bit of core energetic vocabulary, a holophrase, that works to activate your body's miraculous abilities to heal.

HOLOPHRASES

The first words we learn as infants are magical. They are called *holophrases*, which is the use of a single word to express a complex idea. To a young child, *up* refers to much more than a direction. It implies wanting to be picked up or held. The child wants help getting to face level with adults. *Mama* is not just a name for a person; *Mama* is the source of food and comfort, the child's home base. Similarly, saying *ba* for blanket embraces all the importance of this comforting, beloved, snuggly experience. It can also be used as a request — "I want my ba" — or an expression of appreciation: "I love my ba."

Too often when we learn energy modalities, we don't establish this vital level of communication, this personalized baseline vocabulary. Instead we are taught in a more abstract, intellectual way. Theory and practice are focused on what technique to use for what problem. That is the medical model: What's wrong and how can I fix it? Or we learn energy exercises by rote and don't always know how to apply them for our own self-care.

If you build your energy language from the ground up, in the context of dialoguing with your own energies about present conditions and concerns, they will show you what you need in order to thrive.

It is extremely helpful to build up a set of holophrases as you learn energy medicine: Find gestures, touch, images, colors, breathing patterns, and more that bring you home, that encapsulate your most cherished truths, and that represent your ability to name and call in aspects of experience that are important to you. In this and the next two chapters, we will explore how to do this, before launching into more complex and technical kinds of communication in later chapters.

ENERGY VOCABULARY: TOUCH

We are blessed with so many ways of communicating with our subtle energies that it truly is a multidimensional language. The key vocabulary you can use in dialoguing with the energies that make you up includes: touch; gesture; imagery, symbols, and visualization; light and color; sound and rhythm; movement; breath; shapes; scent and taste; intention that helps guide behaviors of subtle energies; and field energies and environmental placement.

When Mother Teresa stepped up to help the man in extreme spasms (which I describe on page 13), she chose touch and rhythm as her modes of communication. The video of this is both jarring and poignant. First, the man she was helping was a member of the untouchable class. Second, she was a nun, not a nurse or doctor, so she was not someone you would expect to intervene by stroking a man's body. Third, she was a stranger who was daring to use touch, when in many cultures touch is reserved for people we know.

But Mother Teresa's choice was brilliant and deeply appropriate to the situation. Touch is our birthright. It can be profoundly healing, yet it is barely part of any medical intervention these days.

Touch is important to our function as creatures. We use touch to communicate with infants, to console children, to connect with friends and lovers. Touch speaks to our Earth Elemental Self and through that to our emotional, thinking, Talking Self. Touch allows energy to transfer or connect, calm or augment, reorganize or disaggregate. Touch can bring you home to yourself or bring you out of a locked-in configuration. I believe it is a primary communication device built into our human instrument. Yet how many people, when asked what their communication apparatus is, would include their hands in the list?

Most of us don't think of using touch to heal ourselves. If I have a headache, I am socialized to think of popping a pill rather than putting my hands on my head, my neck, my body, and using them to calm and release the logjam. Since we live in an extremely touch-phobic society, many of us are also afraid to use touch or are forbidden to use it without a *license to touch*. In most US states, it is illegal to touch people professionally without a massage or medical license. Teachers, pastors, caregivers, therapists, and others whose job it is to console and support people are prevented from using this most basic of equipment because touch in our society has been so distortedly linked to sex.

Your hands communicate with your subtle energies, and with the energies of other people, using the language of energy. It's not something we teach children to understand, though in some cultures they do. Can you imagine raising a daughter (or son) who would automatically use her hands to console herself, to speak to her owies, to shift her energies when they got off-balance, to adjust muscles when they got too tight, to readjust bones and cartilage that got knocked askew, to activate and accelerate healing of wounds or injuries, and to adjust tension, blood pressure, and other bodily functions upward or downward as needed? These are all possible, even easy, to do using your hands.

Most people at least use touch vocabulary in minimal ways: putting your hand to your heart, mouth, or forehead when upset; squeezing a tight shoulder to invite release. Because of that, it is possible to gain fluency in it, even as an adult.

How often and how do you touch yourself? Is it loving communication? I had to teach myself to mother myself with my hands. I grew up pinching unwanted parts of me, wishing they were smaller, flatter, prettier, not there, but not lovingly cradling my physical being.

• • • PLAY WITH IT • • •

Because our society has such a skewed perception of touch, it is important that you develop your holophrases of touch *in private* at first.

How touchy-feely are you already? If you have the habit of touching yourself for various purposes, this exploration will be easy. If not, you may find it more challenging. I scaffolded on what I had learned from petting my cats and dogs. I learned to calm myself by stroking behind my ears and to open up my hearing by pulling on my ears. I stroked my tailbone and imaginary tail to compliment myself; I rubbed my belly to tell myself I was a good girl.

Play with touching yourself — first, to console or calm yourself. It helps if you can bring to mind a situation where you feel upset or else respond to an existing signal of discomfort or need from your body. Then experiment with different types of touch to see what feels helpful and calming. If you are a parent, you can draw on touch you have used with your children.

What are some of the situations in which you might want to communicate via touch with your Earth Elemental Self? Here are some that come to mind:

- To get out of your head and into your heart or gut
- To console yourself when upset
- To come home to yourself
- To calm yourself when overexcited
- To express love
- To make yourself feel heard or listened to
- To clear blockage
- To stimulate energy to flow when you're feeling stuck or dull
- To energize yourself and support yourself to *dare*

- To make yourself feel safe
- To tell yourself nourishment is on its way or to make yourself feel that you are being fed and cared for
- To connect parts of yourself that don't feel like they are communicating
- To help your tired self to relax and let go
- To affirm your pride or satisfaction in a job well done

As you go through the next weeks, practice using touch to speak to your creature self. See what emerges as your core vocabulary or experiment to invent something that works for you.

• • • • • •

Let Creativity and Intuition Guide Your Hands

Let creativity and intuition flow when learning to speak energy with your hands. Letting your body activate that knowing is easier than trying to memorize which touch speaks to which emotions. It doesn't matter if you have the correct touch — the important part is to let yourself intuitively dialogue with energies, letting your hands do the talking.

For example, I find myself getting stressed when I know my cousin is visiting. I like her, but we were very competitive when we were kids, so whenever I'm about to see her, I get anxious. I want to overeat, I notice I'm not breathing very deeply, and I feel like a lump. So I let my hands just initiate dialogue. I start petting my head, like I would pet my dog, including pulling and extending my long doggy ears. That makes me realize how tight my head is. So I pet it a while, then tap my scalp all over to just stimulate energy to move. I feel like I need to pull all that loosened energy out of my head, so stroking downward, I pull it down my whole body and off the ends of my toes. Then I throw it in a universal recycling bin because, if I don't want it, I don't want it cluttering my house.

Then I realize I just want to be held. So I wrap my arms around myself and rock. I grab a large stuffed animal we keep around for the grandkids (official excuse), and hug it for a while, trying to wordlessly communicate consolation to the stuffy. I let myself feel both the mother in me consoling the stuffy and myself as the stuffy receiving that mothering.

I find myself circling my solar plexus with one hand in a counter-clockwise motion, spiraling out into my energy field then back in again, feeling it release energy. Then, without making a conscious decision to do so, I find myself tapping on my chest, like an ape, as if to say: *I am the champ!* I end the conversation by drawing hearts all over my body. Now, when I think about my cousin coming, I feel calm and slightly amused. The desire to chow down on treats has dissipated, and I can tune in to my stomach and notice I'm not hungry.

Remember all the different styles of touch available to you: tapping, stroking, kneading, pulsing, holding, tracing shapes, pulling, pressing, and more. Over time you will find yourself combining the tools — touch plus tapping in rhythms, touch plus using sound, touch plus color, as if your fingers are paintbrushes bringing beauty to all parts of your body. If you are engaging in an actual energetic dialogue and focused on something you care about, you will find yourself able to feel what makes the most difference, rather than just randomly playing with touch.

• • • EXERCISE: HEALING HANDS • • •

Rub your two hands together to activate their healing capacity. You may want to experiment with holding them just an inch or two apart, palms facing each other, to see what you feel radiating from them: Heat? Tingling? Pulsing?

Then take one lovely, healing hand (either left or right), and let it move to wherever on your body it wants to go. Place it, palm facing the skin, on that part of your body. Experiment with what pressure feels right: solid touch, medium touch, light touch? Go with how it feels and try to listen to your body rather than guiding this activity with your mind.

Leave that hand in place, and take your other healing hand and let it move to where it wants to sit, palm down, on your body.

Just hold these two places until one hand gets called to move to another spot. Shift that hand. Then check in with the other hand: Does it want to move somewhere else or stay put?

There is no rule about how long to hold or where to place your hands. Just follow their wisdom, the inclinations of the quiet still voice within, and let yourself feel whatever sensations arise as you use your healing hands.

Continue shifting each hand as it is pulled or guided by your body's wisdom to move. At some point, you will have a sense of completion, that whatever needed to happen has been accomplished for now.

It is fine to do this exercise fully dressed, but it is also lovely to do it in the bath or bed, making contact between your hands and skin. Your body will give you feedback on what it needs each time. And your healing hands will engage in an energetic dialogue your body needs, even when your conscious mind is not able to guide you.

• • • • • •

GESTURE

Before verbal language develops, young children communicate using other kinds of vocabulary, such as sound and movement. Gesture (including facial expressions) is a communication that we instinctively understand and begin to develop very early. That is why parents in many parts of the world teach their babies sign language to express basic desires: More. Enough. Eat. Love. This helps reduce frustration because babies can then communicate needs long before they are capable of speaking.

I saw this basic gestural language reemerge in my grandfather, who was senile in the final three years of his life. He lost his ability to use words with clear purpose, often saying random one- or two-word phrases that clearly did not match what his formerly rapier-sharp brain would have chosen. What began to emerge was a Grandpa R. sign language. If he was frustrated, he would take his hand and strike downward with it, like slapping a tabletop. If he was unhappy, his hand would move from side to side, often accompanied by sounds of distress. If he was upset, he fingered his sleeve and rubbed the fabric.

His caregiver was initially frustrated that Grandpa could no longer tell her what he needed. But eventually she learned to read the signals he *was* capable of using, instead of insisting he find his disappeared words. Toward the end of his time, his caregiver became his interpreter for the family: "He is happy to see you." "He's tired now." "He likes that music."

• • • PLAY WITH IT • • •

Take a moment to experiment with and explore your own "sign language." Practice talking with your hands, body movements, facial expressions, sounds, and any other physical elements you want to bring in. Do this exercise in private and in a place where you have some room, so that you can include dance steps, rhythms, and sounds while using the whole space. *Play* with this exercise and you will get more out of it!

I call this "fake sign language," one that develops your own private code. This is not meant to mimic or disrespect speakers of American Sign Language (ASL) or other formulated gestural languages. This is an exercise in relearning how to communicate through gesture. In fact, if you are a dancer or artist, you probably already do something similar. For dancers, it involves dancing what you feel, expressing your inner truth, nonverbally and without conscious thought, through the medium of movement. Visual artists might recognize it as gestural doodling, letting your hands express feelings through movement and color on the page.

To begin, ask yourself, *How do I feel?* Turn your thinking brain off; it doesn't need to invent something. Let your body just move to answer that question. When it winds down its response, you might also ask, *What do you need in this moment?* Let your body respond organically. Stay open to just letting your creature self express what it wants to, rather than trying to ask pointed questions and looking for pointed answers. Then express yourself using fake sign language.

Example: When I ask myself how I feel, my hands immediately start moving like windshield wipers that are operating appositionally instead of in sync. They are also flailing like someone who can't coordinate her limbs. I realize I'm feeling a kind of alarmed frustration. So I ask myself: *What do you need in this moment?* After a brief pause, my hands start weaving in and out with each other in interlocking figure eights. It is a pattern I call the "Celtic Weave," after an Eden Energy Medicine exercise, but it is not a conscious choice. My hands just choose that gesture from the library in my head. After a few minutes, I ask myself once again: *How do you feel?* Now my hands gently circle around each side as I inhale and move down the center of my body, palms facing the ground, with an audible exhale, as if I am grounding my breath. When I ask myself what I want to say to my body, both hands land on my heart, right over left.

● ● ● ● ● ●

Private Code

Fake sign language can help you attune to some of your core expressive vocabulary. It doesn't need to be something other people can understand. It taps into your own inner library of movements, gestures, sounds, and meaning. It uses your *private code*. The term *private code* is used to refer to private language that can develop between twins, or others who are close, but it also can apply to a private language we develop with ourselves: gestures, sounds, colors, and elements that capture or encapsulate our core *meaning*. Some of these elements may be instinctual, others are built up with experience over time, and others invented to address a need. Activating the private code is often a direct and powerful way to communicate in a vital connection with your own energies.

Janine grew up in a chaotic household with two alcoholic parents. She became the hyper-responsible family member, the one who felt she needed to hold everything together for her parents and siblings. It propelled her onto a path of overachievement: She got three higher degrees in two different fields; she was often the youngest to reach milestones; and she was considered most likely to succeed by her fellow students.

But as she got older, she was aware that behind her supercompetent exterior, she was running way too many stress hormones. She could feel the panic and noticed that if any little thing went wrong, her body reacted as if it was a life-or-death crisis, even as her very capable mind could triage and recognize that little thing as a bump in the road.

Eventually she collapsed and was diagnosed with chronic fatigue.

Looking from the outside, it is easy to see what kind of toll having to hold it together took on Janine. But she had constructed her identity around seeing herself as someone who was born organized, born to achieve, born to lead. She was surprised when she began to dialogue with her body and let it show her what it wanted. After a few sessions playing with fake sign language and dialoguing with her body, she realized she didn't feel safe. She was terrified all the time.

Janine decided she needed a secret signal to let her body and childself know they were protected, even when she was out and about in public. With a little experimentation, she found that if she gently and subtly stroked the inside of her wrist, then drew hearts over it, it would calm the panic and communicate safety. She used this signal extensively when at home, and she discovered that her body would recognize even a subtle version of it when she was at a meeting or getting triggered at the grocery store. Instinctively, she chose a place on her body that corresponds to the meridian responsible for protecting the heart!

Janine went on to develop a number of personalized signals for speaking to her body; she recognized that the terror and sense of danger needed to be addressed immediately when they arose. She also sought out an energy psychologist to help her use meridian tapping (a form of communicating with the body's energy flows) to try to clear experiences from her past that were bleeding through into the present. Within about six months, her fatigue was gone, and she reported that the volume of her body's reactivity was turned way down from her former feelings of panic to a quiet message of "pay attention here." Her body was learning to trust that a responsible adult was on duty and would respond moment by moment to keep her safe.

Private code is not just a vocabulary list of personalized gestures and movement. It is a baseline expression of what is important to you, of meaning. Although you can learn a rich vocabulary of exercises and techniques to speak to the established energy pathways when you study various energy medicine modalities, it is also useful to be willing to invent vocabulary as needed. Your private code energy language allows you to affirm your soul's truth and make quick and direct adjustments to your subtle energies in alignment with your deeper intention.

Experiment with finding gestures (or movements) that help you feel the following energies: opening, connection, flow, metabolizing (or taking stuff in), release, plugging into self and Source, grounding your energies, safety, and communion. We will explore these energies later in the book.

• • • EXERCISE: CABINETS OF WONDERS • • •

Sometimes the body's *gatekeeper* (the part of you that maintains your identity and immune functions; see page 136) will close down a whole area of the energy field, like putting part of your energy body in lockdown. When that happens, energies in that area can be sluggish or just feel stuck. Energy lockdown can also show up as chronic health issues or injury in an area or overall tightness and muscle tension. I call this phenomenon "locking the cabinets of wonders." Imagine your body as a storage place for the creative expressions of your soul in the physical dimension. When these storage places get locked down, your creative juices and everyday functions just can't flow.

Imagine that your pelvic bowl is one such area of great treasures. In many energy traditions, this is the area of the first and second chakras, spinning energy distribution centers that often represent creation, pro-creation, and authentic self. If, for some reason, it does not feel safe for those energetic centers to be open to the energies of others (or the world at large), your body's gatekeeper shuts the cabinet doors and sometimes locks them. This is self-protective but also self-limiting.

The four places you will commonly find locked cabinets are:

1. around the pelvic bowl (protecting your root)
2. around your belly and solar plexus area (the belly button and third chakra, often representing links to nourishment, identity, and creation of self in the world)
3. around the heart and upper rib cage area (protecting the heart, lungs, and back door of the heart)
4. around the head and neck (protecting the head, face, throat, and communications of the mind/spirit)

To open your cabinets, first unlock any locks you sense on the cabinet doors. I usually imagine them as the latches you find in hotel rooms. To open them, first inhale, and then on the exhale, flip them open with a gesture. If you see them as keyed locks, use gesture to insert an imaginary key and turn it.

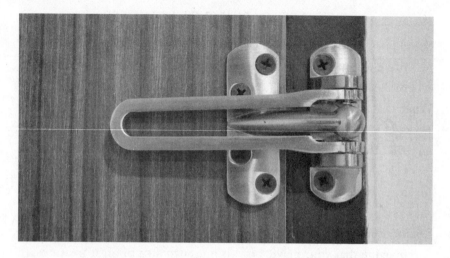

Figure 1. Latch

Then place your two hands flat on the cabinet doors, as if you are inside the cabinet and the doors are in front of you. On the exhale, slowly push the cabinet doors open by spreading your two hands outward, miming the opening of cabinet doors. You can open each of the four cabinets in turn.

Tune in to see what differences you feel when you open your cabinets of wonders.

• • • • • •

IMAGERY, SYMBOLS, AND VISUALIZATION

You can use images, symbols, and visualization to move energies. That is why so many healing modalities rely on the mind to guide healing.

I met Xena early in my training as a medical intuitive. My chiropractor colleague asked me if I could come to her office to meet with a client whose body wasn't responding to treatment. In those days, my inner teachers would often suggest I bring props to the session. For Xena's session, they asked me to bring an orange rubber ball.

It turned out that Xena's blood pressure levels were chronically through the roof and had not responded to medications or nutritional supplements. Xena had sought out the chiropractor to explore possible natural solutions. She was interested in getting pregnant, but her doctor had told her it would not be safe until she brought her blood pressure down.

I was sitting there thinking, *Hmmm, blood pressure....I don't know anything about it. What am I doing here?* I was squeezing the orange ball, wondering if I'd brought it to relieve my own stress and panic, when Xena saw the ball and asked, "What's that for?"

"Good question," I said. "Let's experiment with it. What would your ideal blood pressure numbers be?"

"One-twenty over seventy-five."

"Okay, why don't you throw it up in the air a hundred and twenty times and then bounce it on the ground seventy-five?" Clearly, I was improvising.

Xena was a good sport, so she dutifully did her 120 tosses and 75 bounces. Then the three of us just looked at one another. What now? The chiropractor said, "Well, let's recheck her blood pressure to see if anything shifted." It now registered exactly 120 over 75, which was down from 200 over 120 a few minutes earlier!

We all started laughing because — how ridiculous was that? The chiropractor asked me, "Do you know why that happened?"

Xena said: "I know." She had been in a toy store earlier that week with her partner and their young son. While they were shopping, she picked up an orange ball and started playing with it. Then a somewhat officious salesperson came up to her and asked her to either buy the ball or stop playing. Xena felt deep shame and put the ball back, then she quickly left the store and waited for her family down the street.

"I felt so happy when I was just tossing the ball, remembering how much fun it was when I was a kid. And then the salesperson came and yelled at me, and it never occurred to me I could just buy the ball. I felt I should not be playing!"

Xena's sky-high blood pressure was not just in reaction to her high-stress job as a lawyer but to the fact that her soul was yearning to play. There was not enough permission in her life, from herself and others, to feel she had the right to it. I gave her the ball as a gift and invited her to start welcoming play back into her day-to-day life, even when she was at work.

That was the beginning of a process of self-healing that led Xena to explore the whole web of meanings that related to play for her. Play, as a holophrase and as a concept, became her touchstone to healing, and it led her to gradually shift her career from law, which she liked and was good at, to ministry, which she loved.

Xena's health problems — high blood pressure, fertility issues, and digestive complaints — did not respond to either medical or nutritional treatments because what was wrong was an absence of something *right*, something Xena needed in order to have her body stop shouting at her and digging in its heels.

It took some experimentation and a situation in which we were exploring and asking for insights to bring us all to a realization of what her body was communicating.

If I had come in as an expert on blood pressure or a know-it-all psychic, I would probably not have thought about permission to play as the best medicine. If I had tried to step in as a hero — sedating the appropriate meridians, creating temporary relief — I could have short-circuited the communication from her body that was telling her to explore the opportunities and blockage to *play* in her life.

It was a team effort. I was glad to have the medical backup, screening out life-threatening issues, and the chiropractor with her knowledge of supplements and structural issues, and mostly, the client, who was willing to step outside the box and participate in solving her own problems.

Energy Unity

The term I use for an image, exercise, gesture, or theme that moves energy as a unit is *energy unity*. This is an extension of the holophrase concept.

For example, if I get a phone call from a dear friend, hearing her voice can act as an energy unity, shifting my energies from sluggish to sparkling. Energy unities are powerful energy medicine, and they are accessible to you if you are open to finding images, concepts, movements, or signs that allow your energy to transform. The cabinets of wonders I describe above are good examples of energy unities, as was Xena's orange ball. They were not specific energy treatments; they shifted multiple energy systems at once.

Some energy unities have widespread effectiveness. For example, tracing hearts on the body will generally activate heart energy, even though that is not the shape of the anatomical heart. Drawing figure eights will unify energies to balance your yin and yang. Other energy unities are unique to the individual: Not everyone would respond to bouncing an orange rubber ball as Xena's energies did.

Images carry multiple dimensions of meaning. When I ask clients to tune in and see what is there, many will come up with an image or graphic language, perhaps saying, "I feel wrung out." The phrase conjures the image of a cloth twisted to squeeze out all the moisture. I would invite the client to tune in to that image, asking, "What does your wrung cloth need?" Then we come up with a gesture or exercise that responds to the need.

For example, the "Well of Restitution" is an energy unity my inner teachers gave me when I felt wrung out, drained, and had run out of steam. I pictured myself hopping into a large bucket and using a crank to lower myself into a well of restitution. I actually used the motions of cranking and visualized myself dipping lower, the bucket filling, and let the healing waters wash over me and seep into me to reconstitute my energies. That evening I took a physical bath to make the experience of rehydrating feel real.

Interpretation or Dialogue

An image is not just a mental picture: It is a mental picture that acts as a holophrase, encapsulating meaning. You can approach this in two ways:

1. Unpack the meaning and *interpret* the image.
2. Stay within the language of the image and *dialogue* with it

symbolically: Turn it into a mental video, evolving the energies into a new form.

I often do both. In my self-healing, I find that visualization is even better when accompanied by actions, gestures, sound effects, touch, and feeling each step of the transformation.

Example: I have been suffering from a chronic low-grade sore throat for a few months. I'm not sick, but my throat feels somewhat shredded. When I tune in, I see hanging strands, the image of vertically shredded tissue. I can *interpret* the image: Somehow my life has gotten too linear; I need the warp of my life to have a better woof! And I can use that interpretation to explore what a better woof might look like: Getting to the pool more often? Going for rambling walks? Taking time for non sequiturs and fluff activities? Or maybe I literally need a puppy (*woof-woof*), since sometimes the mind uses images in a punning way!

But I can also *dialogue* with the image by using my fingers to weave some new horizontal strands into the hanging strands at the throat. I don't know consciously what specific strands are needed, so I let my fingers stream all colors of the rainbow. I weave in and out between the vertical strands of shredded tissue with these beautiful horizontal streams. I realize the warp isn't anchored at the base of my throat; the vertical strands I am seeing in my mind's eye look like they are just dangling there. So I take each one, seven in all, and anchor them into my collarbone using pegs, like the tuning pegs on a violin. Now my throat feels anchored, and the beautiful fabric I have created looks a little like a stylized dream catcher.

Time will tell whether this is enough of an energy unity to move the energies and heal my throat. The pain lifts in the moment, so I stop. I can keep exploring the theme that emerged, strengthening the woof, and I will also keep dialoguing and letting the energies show me the way.

LIGHT AND COLOR

Some of my clients, when asked to tune in and see what's there, see colors, shapes, and patterns, but no specific imagery. Color and light can be a baseline vocabulary to play with on their own terms.

Many authors have written books describing the colors of the energy body, detailing what color each chakra is and what it means. (A chakra is a swirling spinning disk of energy that carries subtle energies into and out of the body and its surrounding energy field.) But Donna Eden, who has seen subtle energies in glorious detail her entire life, teaches that from her perspective, those generalized color attributions don't hold true.[3] Each person has an individual mix of colors and patterns of light in each of their chakras and throughout their energy body. And those colors and lights, and geometric shapes and pattern, tell their own unique story. It is probably best to develop your use of color through experimentation, just as you would if you were a painter.

What does that particular shade of green mean to you? How does it make you feel? What happens to your feelings about it if you muddy the color or make it more intense, darken it or lighten it? Green doesn't have the same emotional impact for each person, so although there may be some universal associations built into our creature instincts (associating green with growing things, for example), other common associations, such as envy, are culturally learned.

Matisse encouraged artists to develop their own color palette and their own gestural language, a set of colors and brushstrokes and shapes that form their artistic idiom. This is a great concept for self-healing as well.

Colors are energy, vibrations of light, and as such, they matter. But the particular vibration you crave relates both to what your body's energies are doing and to your associations with the color. If you try to google the symbolic meanings of colors — thinking, *I need grounding*, and looking for the color the experts say is grounding — this will not always communicate what you want.

As kids, most of us were taught to paint a tree trunk brown, the leaves green, the apples red, and the sky blue. Your tree might be more powerful in purple, with polka-dot leaves, orange apples, and a sky of pale yellow! It can be a healing energetic liberation to let your visual vocabulary evolve primarily in reference to your own feelings, rather than in lockstep with cultural thoughts.

• • • PLAY WITH IT • • •

Tune in to an area of your body that needs some attention. Ask what it needs. An infusion of light? Does it want a particular color? Use your fingers as paintbrushes, or your palms as light sources, to bring color or light into that area.

Sometimes, if the area won't accept the light or color, it is helpful to start by working with the color that is already there. Place your hand over the area and use your inhale to bring a new shade in; for instance, lighten the black to a dark purple, then use your exhale to help the new shade to integrate and distribute through the area. Shade by shade, you can gradually support the transformation in that area to the color it seems to want.

There is no need to fear color and light work. Sometimes an area will say it wants to go darker, toward absence of color. That can actually be quite restful. Pay attention to how it feels and use those feelings as a guide. Just as putting yourself in darkness is sometimes the best way to recover from a migraine, sometimes the body needs to remove the light and color for a time to generate new light and patterns.

• • • • • •

• • • EXERCISE: THE FOUR STABILIZING COLORS • • •

An excellent technique to stabilize any area of work, or the whole body, is to use the Four Stabilizing Colors. This pattern was given to me by an inner teacher who had a somewhat shamanic style of healing. The four colors can be seen as stations on a flow wheel (see figure 2).

Using the four corners of the torso (front of right hip, front of right shoulder, front of left hip, front of left shoulder), place either hand flat on each position, starting with the front of the right hip and the color yellow. Imagine your body and entire field filling with *yellow* light.

When you feel full, move your hand to the second position, front of right shoulder, and imagine your body and aura filling with *red* light.

When that is full, move to position three, front of left shoulder, place your hand flat, and imagine your body and aura filling with *black* light, the darkness of the night sky.

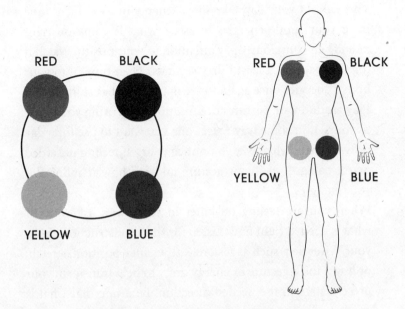

Figure 2. The Four Stabilizing Colors

When that is full, move to position four, front of left hip, place your hand flat, and imagine your body and aura filling with *blue* light.

You can use these four colors to stabilize an organ by using the corresponding four corners of the organ area (imagine laying the diagram on the area to determine which corner is which).

It can also be used as a meditation, or done using colored light or colored gauze you shine light through.

• • • • • •

PRACTICE TIPS

- When you don't know what you need, and can't hear your subtle energies communicating, use the "Healing Hands" exercise (page 74). Turn off your brain and let your hands do the talking. This is a great go-to communication when your brain or senses are unclear about what to do.

- Throughout your day, take short "energy breaks." First, tune in to your subtle energies to assess what is going on right *now*. Then consciously pay attention to your breath. Watch it for the space of at least thirty seconds. Then tune in to your body's energies once again to see if anything has shifted.

- Play around with gestures or sensations that bring you home to yourself in some way. Select one you want to use for a day or two. Then, whenever you notice yourself feeling unsettled or off-balance, use your gesture and see how it influences your energies.

- When you are feeling off-kilter in some way, ask yourself what is needed right now. Listen for simple instructions from your Wiser Self, such as rest, release, change position, stretch, or hug. Find a gesture or energy unity to help transform your present state in the needed direction. Be aware that what is needed might not relate directly to what feels off.

- The energy vocabulary for communicating with subtle energies in this chapter can guide explorations over time. Each day, choose one item — touch; gesture; imagery, symbols, and visualization; or light and color — and experiment with how many ways you can use that throughout your day. For example, if you choose touch, explore all the ways you can touch yourself or use touch to communicate with your subtle energies for the space of twenty-four hours. Use this exploration to give you insights into how you already use touch and how you could use it more consciously to communicate with your body.

- Experiment to discover how everyday activities and actions act as an energy unity to shift your overall sense of flow and well-being. What happens to you energetically when you wash dishes, play with the cat, rearrange your spices, doodle, shower, and so on?

- At least once a day, ask your Earth Elemental Self how it is and what it wants from you. Have a conversation with your Earth

Elemental Self using your fake sign language, so you become familiar with this style of dialogue.

- Practice getting information in various ways (through image, sound, feel, smell, and so on) and then both unpack the meaning of the communication *and* dialogue with it to transform the energy.

Chapter Five

THE LANGUAGE OF SOUND, MOVEMENT, AND PATTERN

The subtle energies of the body — and even the energies in an apparently solid object — move in patterns: Energy vibrates in waves, it congregates in fields, it communicates via *resonance* and *influence*. Resonance is when one energy sets another vibrating in attunement, even at a distance. Influence is when the vibration of one energy catalyzes vibration in another.

In this chapter, we'll explore five more ways of communicating with subtle energies: sound, rhythm, movement, breath, and shapes (for the complete list, see page 44). We will work with energy movements and the shapes or patterns that can influence those movements and catalyze change.

SOUND AND RHYTHM

Musick has Charms to sooth a savage Breast,
to soften Rocks, or bend a knotted Oak.

— William Congreve, *The Mourning Bride*, 1697

Sound is a tool we can use to easily and intuitively communicate with our subtle energies via resonance and influence, using vibration, patterns,

91

and fields of sound. You have probably experienced this: Shifts in mood and energy level occur when you hear a lullaby, listen to a favorite song, chant for a few minutes, get lost in an orchestral masterpiece, or overhear a pounding beat in the car next to you at a stoplight!

I remember as a kid trying to replicate the television ad where a soprano hits a high note, causing a crystal glass to shatter. Fortunately, my glass wasn't fine crystal, and my voice, while high, was not powerful enough to shatter glass. But I was successful at finding tones of voice that would annoy my sister, cause my dog to wag her tail and roll over to get her belly rubbed, cajole adults to smile at me, and make friends feel loved. Sometimes I'd find songs that would cause my stomach to stop hurting; cause my sadness to turn liquid, flow out, and release; and encapsulate the joy I felt that no words could express.

Sound is a rich and powerful healing tool, especially for self-healing. Music can be used to create or alter mood, heal the soul, and invoke the sacred, which is a core ingredient in wellness. Music can also be used to move and influence the subtle energies that bathe your organs and run your body's functions.

I am very tonal, which means I process energies using my ears to pick up vibrations, sounds, rhythms, cadences, and tones. And I understand the energies they represent. Being tonal also means I am often driven crazy by sound pollution, such as constant Muzak, background music, the noise of banging machines, the hum of refrigerators and air-conditioning, and the sounds of TV and radio filling all the empty spaces in many settings. If sound has the power to move us and influence our energies, and it does, then the soundscape of contemporary life can easily cause energetic and even stress-chemical overload in people who are sensitive to sound.

Consider: A driving beat in music can get you excited and make you want to jump to your feet and dance. It is a stimulant, causing chemical cascades that can really move you. But too much of that driving beat acts on your body like multiple cups of coffee. Calming classical music, on the other hand, can act to bring your stress hormones down. I once visited a tequila factory that plays classical music 24/7 in the room where the tequila is fermenting to keep the yeast calm and balanced!

Sound healing is vast. Like other energy vocabulary you can use to communicate with your subtle energies, I recommend you experiment and create your own baseline experience with it.

In using sound for self-healing, however, you may need to first clear your palate and experience some silence! I used to go twice a year to ten-day silent meditation retreats in the desert, and while there wasn't total silence, the return to immersing myself in the sounds of nature, unembellished by recorded sound, other people's chatter, and machine noise reset my ability to use sound as a healing tool (for myself and others). If you can't afford this kind of luxury, then an hour or two spent in a park immersed in natural sounds can help clear your instrument.

• • • PLAY WITH IT • • •

Experiment with individual sounds and how they affect you overall. See what types of sounds move you and how. What happens when you sing short notes versus sustained ones?

Find a place in your body that you are drawn to for some reason. Maybe there is pain or congestion there or another sensation that calls your attention. Experiment with sending sound into that area, either by holding your hand there and singing or just by aiming sound toward that area with your intention.

Try *toning*: vocalizing a sound and letting it vibrate through your body. Does it work better to sing the tone clear or with vibrato? Does it work better to hold the note in a sustained way or to use a rhythm with it? What happens when you combine a few notes — does the music want to rise, fall, or perhaps circle around?

Experiment with how it feels in your body to *make* sounds, how it feels to *listen* to sounds, and how it feels to try to *hear sounds with your whole body*. Try visiting a gong store to feel what happens in your subtle energies as you strike different tones; listen to various kinds of sacred chants online to see what effect they have on you. Make up your own sacred chant: Sing your celebration of the Divine in your own made-up chant.

Do these exercises embarrass you? Although our culture is full of sound and noise, we are also all too frequently shamed when using our voices, vocalizing, and expressing ourselves with sound. Because many cultures and subcultures carry a belief that children should be seen and not heard, too many children grow up finding it hard to use sound easily and without self-consciousness. Many of us got shamed if we tried to sing but couldn't carry a tune. Sound that is blocked or unexpressed can cause physical and emotional illness, and people whose voices are chronically silenced by others may suffer chronic illness as a result. Reclaiming sound and finding your voice, both literally and figuratively, is a powerful wellness practice.

• • • • • •

• • • EXERCISE: SIMPLE ENERGY SELF-TEST • • •

Although my emphasis in this book is on tuning in to perceive energies directly, developing some skill with energy testing is useful as well.

This simple Eden Energy Medicine energy self-test, called the Pendulum Self-Test, works on the pendulum principle. Stand up with both feet together, tuck each elbow into your side, with your hands together on your solar plexus, one over the other.

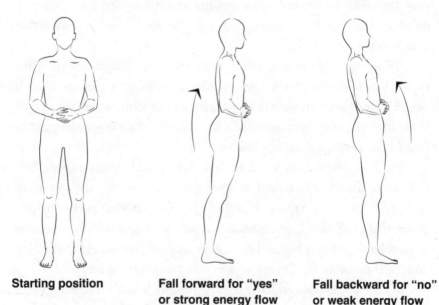

Starting position   **Fall forward for "yes"**   **Fall backward for "no"**
                              or strong energy flow   **or weak energy flow**

Figure 3. Pendulum Self-Test

Sway a bit forward and back, just to feel your balance loosen. Then say something you know to be true: "My name is [Ellen]." Release your standing balance, so your body can sway backward or forward in response to that statement.

Normally, the body sways forward or toward the truth (your yes), and it sways backward or away from something untrue (your no). Occasionally I meet someone for whom this pattern is reversed.

Try a phrase you know to be untrue: "My name is Mergatroyd." Release your standing balance and see which way your body sways.

Once you have calibrated this Pendulum Self-Test to reliably sway in one direction when you state energetic truths, and backward for untruths, you can use it to validate your body-based intuition.

• • • • • •

Rhythm

Rhythm involves organizing sounds into patterns. These patterns affect the pace and movement of your subtle energies, and they also help to support coordination and organization among your energy systems. Trying to live the wrong pace or rhythm can cause illness. A good number of my clients have found that their natural rhythm and pace were slower or faster, smoother or more syncopated, than their workplace or family commitments demanded. The stress of this mismatch not only affected their self-esteem, but it also caused their body functions to go into overdrive, degrade, or shut down.

• • • PLAY WITH IT • • •

Find a place on your body that calls your attention. If you want to integrate energy testing into this exploration, you can energy-test the energies flowing through that area by placing the pads of your fingers, or your thumb and the first two fingers bunched together, on the designated spot. This is called *energy localizing*. Tuck your elbows into your sides and use the Pendulum Self-Test. Find an area to energy-localize where you get a "weak" or "untruth" or "fall back" response. This will be your *pre-test*.

Now, find a rhythm you want to tap on your body. Use your intuition about where you want to do the tapping — it is not necessary to tap on the area you are trying to influence. Tap that rhythm for a while, using your own sense of what you need or letting your hand choose the rhythm.

Then tune in to see how the original area feels. Repeat the pendulum test while energy-localizing the target area to see if you still fall back or whether you now fall forward, indicating a stronger energy flow through the area. This is your *post-test*.

Example: I am drawn to the left side of my neck, where I have chronic tightness in the muscle that sometimes triggers migraines. The muscle feels tight as I energy-localize it, and I get a "weak" or fall-back pendulum test. Something there is not flowing right! I tap a rhythm with my fingertips on my stomach area. That's where my hand wants to tap, and the rhythm my hand falls into is *ta-ta* pause *ta-ta*, with a slight syncopation. I don't consciously figure out that rhythm — it's just what my hand guides me to do. I tap for about thirty seconds on my stomach and notice that my neck now feels looser. My pendulum post-test, when I energy-localize the same spot on my neck I pre-tested, shows a "strong" or falling-forward test, validating that energy is now flowing in that area.

• • • • • •

• • • EXERCISE: CORE NOTE • • •

In chapter 4, I tell the story of Myra, who used her core note to raise her energy levels to cope with a stressful job. Using the core note brings resources up from our deepest levels; it is a very different kind of energetic activation than what you experience when playing stimulating rap music.

Each of us has a core note that corresponds to the energetic grid that serves as the foundation for all our other energies. The core note represents the energetic vibration of your grid. But the core vibration is different in each individual. Each of us is tuned to a key that is specific to our soul's song.

Are there others who have the same core note as you? Absolutely!

When you meet these people, you often recognize something familiar and comfortable about them. On some level, they may feel like a twin or soul mate.

Singing or listening to your core note can strengthen and reinforce your energy foundation. It can also bring you home to yourself, like using a pitch pipe to sound a note and get the whole choir singing in the same key. Singing songs in the key of your core note will balance your energies and often both console and energize you. They can untangle your mind and body energetically! Singing your core note can help you quickly feel grounded, centered, and plugged into a deep source of energy.

You can also use the core note in conjunction with other energy medicine exercises to help your energies organize more quickly and/or hold their balance longer.

Your core note corresponds roughly to a note on the musical scale. But of course, notes vary greatly in pitch and in vibration (measured as hertz), and our measurement system of notes organizes into different octaves. So, to find your core note, I recommend using your own voice to initially locate the note, when possible, rather than using a piano or musical instrument.

Once you have located it, you can name that note by finding the closest approximation on a piano, then identifying whether it runs a bit sharper or flatter than the standard note. You can also buy an inexpensive gadget called a *chromatic tuner* or download a free app (such as Pano Tuner) that will tell you both the measurement in hertz and the name of the note you are singing.

Finding Your Core Note

Start by singing the note that is most comfortable for your voice to sing. That is often your core note. About three in five of my clients find the core note easily this way. I use energy testing to verify whether the note being sung does in fact match the resonance of their grid. Often the clients who easily sing their core note are able to *feel* that it is core. But if you feel doubt, or want verification, use the following self-test.

Place one hand flat on the front of your *left* shoulder and the other hand flat on your *left* pelvic bone. Sing the note most comfortable for you to sing, and use the Pendulum Self-Test (see "Simple Energy Self-Test," page 94). If you aren't sure, you can just sing a variety of notes and energy-test each one.

The core note will cause you to fall backward; all other notes on the scale will cause you to fall forward.

This might seem counterintuitive, since you would think that the core note would cause you to fall toward the truth. Think of this as an exception to the rule: Most people fall backward when encountering the sacredness of their core truth. This is a good example of how energy testing is an art form, not scientific!

Note: Energy testing is well worth learning by studying modalities like Eden Energy Medicine or Touch for Health.[4] In the context of this book, I am only offering the Pendulum Self-Test as a way to occasionally validate your intuition because I want to encourage you to learn energy dialogue more fully through perceiving and attuning to subtle energies using all your senses.

• • • • • •

Using Music to Guide Healing

Because sound is such a primary expression of subtle energy, much of what we know about music can be used as a metaphor or guide in energy healing.

Louise loved music and sang in choirs as a kid. She came to see me because she suspected her marriage was making her sick (chronic nausea, dizziness, and disturbances in her visual field). Her doctor had dismissed her symptoms as not medically significant. We were able to use her sensitivity to music to explore what was happening in her marriage. It was difficult to discuss it directly because every time she talked about her husband she would feel sick.

First, I asked her to sing a note that she felt represented her. That was easy for her. I then asked her to sing a note that represented her husband. She sang another note. As she was singing her husband's note, I sang the one she had identified as hers. It was an awful dissonance! We both burst out laughing, and she said, "I am actually feeling nauseated just doing this exercise."

I invited her to shift her note to something else. Something that was still true for her, but which might go better with her husband's note. (I sang the husband's note so she could experiment.) She found one she liked, and within a few minutes, the nausea cleared up.

At first Louise was upset by this. She asked: "Why should I have to change my note in response to him?" We had her imagine him in various situations: with her stepson; with his mother; relaxing on vacation. Louise sang the note she thought was true of him in each situation. They were not all the same note. We then discovered that if she sang the note she preferred for herself, it harmonized with everything but the note for his mother.

Louise realized what was making her sick. Whenever her husband treated her like his mother, she felt her symptoms.

She went home with the self-care tool of finding a musical antidote whenever he triggered her. She treated her symptoms as red flags that she was feeling like his mother and found ways to address the issue more appropriately in those moments.

MOVEMENT

Here are a few core principles about subtle energies of the body:[5]

- Energy moves constantly — it wants and needs to move.
- Energy needs space to move.
- Energy prefers to move in specific patterns that allow it to get where it needs to go, but it will find alternative (and sometimes highly individualized) paths if it is blocked.
- Blocked energy negatively affects your health, and the health of the body is a reflection of the health of your energies.
- All the body's energies are interconnected.

Even when you are sitting still, your subtle energies are moving. They are swirling, circulating, communicating, and fueling the work of your body, mind, and spirit. And of course, your body itself is moving: Your chest lifts and falls with each inhale and exhale; your blood circulates as the heart pumps; your muscles move and shift in subtle ways to maintain balance and release tension. The synapses of your brain fire constantly, and the electrical messaging travels endlessly via the nervous system to all parts of your body.

You don't need to consciously tell this movement to happen; it is built into the system. But you most certainly will notice if that movement is blocked! Try stopping your breath for a number of seconds. It creates discomfort, panic, and finally a forced gasp. Similarly, your subtle energies will create discomfort, panic, and a forced gasp if they do not have space to move or are diverted from their healthiest patterns of movement.

One of the principles underlying much of Chinese medicine is to support the subtle energies to move the way they are designed to move. This includes the energy flows called *meridians*, the deeper flows called *strange flows* in Chinese medicine (referred to as *radiant circuits* within Eden Energy Medicine), and the five elements that create our balance and flow. Other energy medicine modalities build on that notion as well: clearing the chakra energies and aura so they can do their job; opening space in the body using physical movement and postures; supporting the in-out or yin-yang pumping of the energies; and other core energy movements that have been distorted and are impacting our health and well-being.

Therefore, movement is a key building block of the language of energy. You know this on a practical level. You may be feeling sluggish and tired, but if you get up and stretch, or motivate yourself to go out for a gentle walk or into the pool to stretch your arms and legs, you generally feel better. Like much of the energy medicine you already do, stretching, movement, massaging a tight muscle, and other activities really speak to the subtle energies: You are making room for energy to move and, in some cases, supporting your energies to flow the way they are designed to flow.

Movement is necessary to your health — not structured exercise, not working out, but movement itself. Your lymph system, which is designed to carry toxins out of the body, is the only system meant to circulate in the body that does not have a built-in pump. Movement is its pump. Blood has the heart to pump it, oxygen has the lungs, food waste has the peristalsis of the intestines. But if you want the garbage and toxic waste that is in your blood to move out of your body, you need to pump it via movement.

Therefore, simple movement — even if it is gentle stretching, slow rocking, or tightening and releasing muscles — can help heal many ailments. Learning to support energies to move as they are designed to move affirms a core baseline function that is needed for your body's wonderful healing properties to work.

• • • EXERCISE: GO WITH THE FLOW — THE K-27 THUMP • • •

If you ever find yourself drained rather than energized after a walk, it is most likely because your meridian energies, the energy pathways that feed the work of your organs and muscles, are flowing backward, so you are working against the flow and it depletes you.

Try tapping or thumping two points to get the meridian energies moving forward again: These are the twenty-seventh points on the kidney meridian, located one inch in from the inner edge of the collar bone and one inch down, in between the top and the first rib, in the divots (see figure 4). The K-27 points act as key junctions for the entire meridian flow pattern.

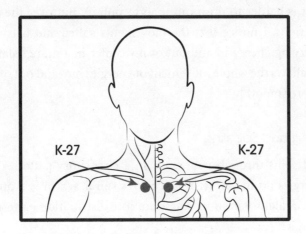

Figure 4. The K-27 points

Tapping helps stimulate energy flow. Try tapping elsewhere on your body to get energies moving there as well.

• • • • • •

Movement Patterns of Subtle Energies

Here are some basic movement patterns of subtle energies for you to explore: in-out, circulating and spiraling, cycling, cross-overs, and figure eights.

In-Out

Both the lungs and the heart have an in-out motion. If you consider them closely, it is not just in-out. The pattern serves a purpose: in, assimilate nutrients; out, distribute nutrients and release waste.

Tune in to how you feel throughout your body. Then use your arms to express in-out movements, finding a rhythm that feels good. Feel into whether one direction is easier than the other, whether you make smooth transitions or feel stickiness at some part of the movement. If you want to align your breathing to the in-out motion, explore what that feels like. Then "freestyle" and *dance* the concept of in-out. Check into your body again once you have finished: What has shifted?

Example: When I do this, I start just pushing and pulling with my arms and find it is harder to push out than to pull in. But over the course of a few rotations, I notice that the movements soften and become figure eights, carrying energy in and out of my center in a more balanced pattern. This allows the whole movement of energies into and out of my body to flow more smoothly.

Circulating and Spiraling

The blood spins through your body in a circulatory pattern. Your meridian energies do the same. Your chakras spiral, which is a progressive, repetitive circulatory motion. These are core distribution patterns for the subtle energies.

Explore making circulatory patterns on your body and in your field. See what it feels like to draw small circles, whole-body circles, and spirals. Circle your arms and legs in various patterns. Feel into what you are saying to your body with your circling motions. What happens when you spiral in or out, up or down, in front or behind you?

Try pulling the energies of the earth up from the ground, over your head, and circulating them down your back to return to the earth. This movement up the front and down the back is the approximate natural path of the meridian energy streams that feed us. Explore what it feels like to use your hands and trace this natural circulation pattern three to five times.

Cycling of Energies

Related to the concept of circling is the cycling of energies. We cycle daily through patterns of sleep and wake; of eating, digesting, and eliminating; of building up and breaking down. We cycle in our moods, energies, and hormones.

• • • EXERCISE: SHIFTING CYCLES • • •

If you can help a particular cycle to keep moving, you can often support all of your body's cyclic processes. Bring to mind a situation that feels off-balance to you right now. It might be something in your health or something in your relationship with another person. Keeping that situation in your mind, make a large circle in the air in front of you to represent the four phases of the moon.

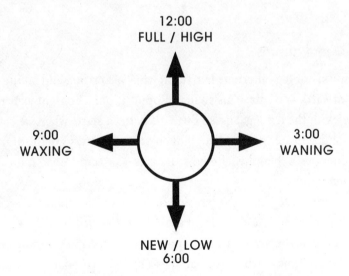

Figure 5. The four phases of the moon

At the bottom of the circle (the six o'clock position on a clock that's facing you) is the new moon or low tide, and as you circle clockwise (moving your hand up on the left to nine o'clock) is the waxing moon, twelve o'clock is the full moon or high tide, and three o'clock is the waning moon.

Circle slowly and see where your hand moves easily and where it stops or requires pressure to continue. Notice where you feel that resistance in the moon's cycle you are drawing. Wherever you feel blockage, stop and draw hearts on that part of the circle, and send love to the situation that is in your mind. Draw hearts on your heart and any other part of your body that feels reactive to the linked issue (head, heart, gut, joints). Then keep moving your arm, bringing love to any part of the cycle that is not moving easily.

Observe the situation you first brought to mind. Have your feelings or the energies shifted? This exercise sometimes takes time to achieve results, but as you become steadier in your larger cycles, your day-to-day experiences evolve.

Symbolic movement can often shift energy patterns that aren't moving easily for us. Not only can symbolic movements help us identify where we are stuck, they can also help us to clear the path so the movement — and energy pattern — can proceed.

• • • • • •

Cross-Over Patterns

As we walk, our legs alternate left/right, while also rising and falling as we move forward, and our arms swing in opposition: The right arm moves forward with the left leg, and so on. This pattern starts when we crawl as infants and activates natural left/right cross-over patterns in the brain and subtle energies. When the left/right energies don't cross over, it is called a *homolateral state*.

In Chinese medicine, the left side of the body is seen as the receptive or "feminine" energy, and the right as the assertive or "masculine" energy. The relationship between these two poles is depicted as a yin-yang symbol of light and darkness, where the light has a little drop of darkness in it, and the darkness a drop of light.

The alternation of left/right, left/right is what moves us forward, and

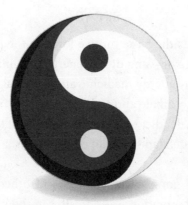

Figure 6. Yin-yang symbol

the action of rising (leaving the earth) and falling (returning to the earth) similarly symbolizes the many ways our energies have tides that rise and fall.

Experiment with motions and movements that alternate left/right or rise/fall. What happens to your energies and mood as you rise, fall, and emphasize left or right? After a time of alternating left/right and rise/fall, check your overall sense of your body. Do you feel different as a result of these movements?

Figure Eights

People who see subtle energies describe the energy field as filled with figure eights of all sizes and moving in all directions. The more figure eights, the healthier the body. These figure eights are part of a larger energy system, called the Celtic Weave, which integrates our various energy flows into harmony. Tracing figure eights in your field, on your body, and every which way is a great tool for supporting integration of your energies literally and figuratively.

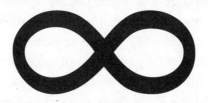

Figure 7. The figure eight

BREATH

The breath represents the basic motive force in the universe, the in-out, *lub-dub*, feed-release, yin-yang of our energetic being. Because of this, it is at the root of many energy medicine and spiritual practices. The word *inspire* means both to inhale and to have your spirit activated. The word *expire* means to exhale, die, give up the ghost. Built into our words for breathing are an understanding that it represents a deep transaction of life and death.

Yoga, tai chi, qi gong, sacred dance, and other healing modalities use breath with great intention. Your breath can show you a lot about how you are taking in, using, releasing, and resting in relationship to your body's energies. And you can use your breath to communicate with your body's energies, to reset the in-out, *lub-dub* necessary for good health.

• • • PLAY WITH IT • • •

Spend a few minutes just watching your breath, without trying to influence it or control it. Is it deep and easy or do you stop yourself on the inhale, cut off the part where your body is using the oxygen, release only partway, or rush into the next breath? Just notice which part of the motion is smooth and which part is challenged. This can actually give you a lot of insight into how you transact with energies across the board.

Experiment with moving your hand, then repeating the motion, but this time correlating it with an inhale, then an exhale. What happens when you correlate your breathing with the movement?

In a lot of my energy medicine exercises, I use the breath to help move energy, inhaling to bring the energy in or activate it, exhaling to help power a shift or to guide a release. It is not necessary to correlate breath with movement, but I find it is often helpful.

Find a place on your body where you are experiencing pain or tightness. Putting one hand there to guide your attention, send your breath into the area. Experiment with whether it wants the inhale or the exhale energy or both. You might even want to put some energetic medicine into the breath: Fill it with love, forgiveness, compassion, or even an energetic painkiller. All medicine is a form of messaging. The breath, fascia, and water are all excellent carriers of energetic messaging.

Experiment with two patterns: (1) Inhale peace, exhale stress; and (2) inhale stress, exhale peace. Both of these can help you move toward peace and release.

Practice this for several minutes, then stop to investigate whether the pain has shifted.

• • • • • •

SHAPES

Subtle energy needs anchors to root it in our shared reality and containers to give it shape and form.

The subtle energies are organized and, in a sense, both anchored and contained by shapes. Like bones that give shape to the viscera and flesh of the body, these geometric shapes help subtle energies to maintain their integrity and flow. Some of these shapes are individual, and others are universal. For example, a whole-body diamond is a pattern that can be seen in most people. On the other hand, we each have at least one core shape (see page 109) that is an organizing factor unique to us.

Terry was a client who needed work with shapes, anchors, and containers because her life was spinning out of control. Her partner was talking about leaving her, complaining she was always in a crisis. She felt disoriented, had difficulty sleeping, and was putting on weight. Her doctor found nothing wrong. At work, she often had to spend hours redoing assignments after making careless errors. She had trouble staying on task.

Her decline began after a four-day vision quest class she took a year earlier. In this class, they did some preliminary exercises, rituals, and meditations, heard talks on vision quests, and spent a little time preparing a small backpack of necessities. Then they were taken out into a wilderness area, each on their own, to quest for vision.

Terry had loved the class, feeling it would help her deepen her spiritual practice and understanding. She desperately wanted to meet her spirit guides and awaken to her warrior self, as the advertisements for the class had suggested. But she was disappointed with the vision quest experience. She did her best to stay open, but the night frightened her. Being alone out in nature made her feel unsafe rather than strong.

Terry diligently practiced the techniques she had been taught, and she kept pushing her mind and consciousness to expand, to take in the unseen world around her. Yet her body pushed back, trying to force her to sleep, shut down, tune out. The only spirit guide she met was a vole, sitting on her backpack in the morning, when she woke up after hours of uncomfortable struggle and only one hour of sleep.

At first, Terry shrugged the experience off. Apparently, though, her body did not. Shortly after that weekend, the sleep difficulties and distraction at work began. Her heart would race, then she'd drop into lethargy. She started to feel criticized every time her partner spoke to her.

When I tuned in to Terry's energies, I felt little flames flaring out, little waves of panic or reactivity. Her aura (energy field) was huge and too permeable, as if she had broken the container that held her energies together. It appeared that in her desire to open to spiritual wisdom, she had somehow breached the natural boundaries of self that were built into her gatekeeper, the part of her consciousness designed to maintain an identity (for more on this, see chapter 7). By trying to open it so quickly and intensively, she had caused her gatekeeper to go into a panic, and it was alternately trying to please her by expanding and keep her safe by shutting her down.

It was clear she needed to reestablish her containers because she was getting buffeted by every energy she encountered.

We explored shapes she could use as energetic containers that would reassure her gatekeeper while still allowing her to let in spiritual influence. These shapes included her core shape (see page 109), a large diamond, and a five-pointed star from her preferred spiritual tradition representing the balance of five elements: air, fire, earth, water, and spirit.

Terry practiced drawing these shapes around and all over her body. She could feel them bring her back into focus. That was her self-care task: to use the shapes and hold off for a time on pursuing her quest to open. Within a month, her sleep and eating patterns had returned to normal, and her work and relationship had improved considerably. Over time, she was able to find a spiritual mentor to guide her on a more gradual path to awakening.

• • • EXERCISE: CORE SHAPE • • •

Your core shape can bring you back into alignment with your own physical being. It helps your body's energies to communicate better, calming your immune system.

Your core shape is like the core note — it sets the pattern for who you are. It is a shape found throughout your subtle energy field and body, down to the cellular level. When you trace this core shape, it reinstates your baseline energies and brings you home to your individuality: It promotes wellness specific to your soul's truth.

There are a number of ways to find your core shape. First, spend about five minutes just doodling. Don't guide the doodle with your brain, but let your hand move, as if you were doodling in a meeting or during a phone call. Then look over your doodle: Is there a recurring shape or pattern on the page that particularly speaks to you?

Core shapes are usually basic, like a circle, rectangle, triangle, pyramid, or hexagram. Or they can be a bit more ornate, like three circles together, a spiral, or a starburst.

Ask your Wiser Self for guidance in recognizing your core shape and pay attention to shapes around you. Which ones do you feel most drawn to?

Use the Pendulum Self-Test to verify whether the shape you are drawn to is in fact your core shape. Stand with your feet together, elbows tucked to your sides, and draw the shape on your solar plexus or belly area with a *three-finger notch*: your index finger, middle finger, and thumb bunched together. Keep in mind that you are looking for your core shape. Do you fall toward it or away?

As with the core note, you generally will fall away from your core shape, but toward other shapes your body likes.

Note: It is not cheating to just take a guess at your core shape and use it all day, tracing it over parts of your body. See if it has a positive effect. If not, try a different shape the next day, until you find one that consistently brings you home to yourself in some way. The good news is that tracing most shapes will bring some benefit because they will reinforce the natural movements of your subtle energies.

For example, Samantha found her core shape by doodling. It was a triangle, and she found through experimentation that it often felt better to trace the triangle and then trace a circle around it. She used this tool intensively for a week; it made her feel more present in her body. But she also felt a need to sink it deeper inside. She laid out a large triangle surrounded by a circle in her yard and walked that pattern: first the triangle, then the clockwise circle. She found it put her into a deep meditative state and opened her to inner guidance. She used it at the beginning and end of each day to create an individualized container for that day's experiences, and she found it helped her to start her day in a more centered way and to sleep more deeply at night.

• • • • • •

PRACTICE TIPS

- Pay attention to the role that sound plays in your day and ask yourself how sound is affecting you. Is there a soundtrack that you have chosen, or that others, including your living space, are imposing on you? What happens to your body or energies in response to the sounds around you. Can you use sound more purposefully to support your body to establish what feels like healthy patterns?

- Use your body like a drum to figure out what rhythm matches your most comfortable energetic pace and beat. When life gets over- or underwhelming, or just in moments of transition (in the morning, at night, when shifting tasks), tap that rhythm on your body to bring you home to yourself and reset your energies to your default. What pace and rhythms best represent your workplace, your home, the people you are closest to? Being conscious of rhythms, and using them with purpose, helps you to affirm your own nature, while accommodating to the demands of your life.

- Find moments of silence throughout your day — stilling even the voices in your head and just tuning in to the sounds of your breath. These moments will act as sorbet to clear your palate.

- Practice using the pendulum energy self-test to check your intuitive hits and to become more accurate when asking your body for feedback. It is well worth the effort to get comfortable with this tool.
- Use your core note and core shape in an ongoing way to build your inner strength and bring resilience to your energetic core. They support your deepest energy systems and give your subtle energies a baseline to organize around.
- When you are feeling symptoms, experiment with the various movement patterns presented in this chapter to see what your body needs in order to support your subtle energies.

Chapter Six

THE LANGUAGE OF INSTINCT, INTENTION, AND PLACEMENT

Despite our evolved and complex culture, we are still creatures of nature, albeit domesticated ones! But like dogs and cats (and wild animals), you can use those creature instincts built into you for communicating and healing. Animals sniff and taste things to get information; they signal with scent, mark their territory, and respond strongly to the environment. We do, too, though not always in ways we recognize. As we have evolved, we have added choice and intention as energetic tools. These can help you to shape your reality beyond the creature patterns coded into your Earth Elemental Self.

SCENT AND TASTE

At Celestial Seasonings, one man has worked as their primary tea tester for over forty years. His sense of smell and taste are so refined that he can sip or sniff a cup of tea and tell you which ingredients are in it. Similarly gifted people work in the wine, cheese, and fine food industries.

Scent communicates with the subtle energies and can influence mood, chemical messaging, and motivation. Taste has similar properties.

Homeopathic remedies, essential oils, Bach flower remedies, foods, spices, and scented items all offer energy vocabulary that can activate or transform our subtle functions.

Andrea was having serious mood swings. These were not just variations between high and low, but feelings that were all over the map: cravings, aversion, excitement, alarm, amazement. She described it as having full-time PMS.

When I checked an energy feature I call the *four burners* (see the exercise "Adjusting the Flames," page 115), which influences both hormones and immune system reactivity, they were all fluctuating erratically. They looked like candle flames dancing in swirling winds.

I suspected Andrea was reacting to subtle stimulants rather than suffering primarily from a hormone problem. Energy testing scents and tastes verified that. She brought a selection of scents and foods she typically encountered in her day. We did a few preliminary energy exercises to balance her energies and then set her four burners to moderate levels with steady flames.

One by one, she then sniffed or tasted each item she had brought to test. She would tune in to her flames and to her emotions and moods to see if they had shifted. Then we verified her perceptions using energy testing.

We discovered that almost any scent that was not related to food would trigger her. Some of the foods would also set her flames flickering and fluctuating, with accompanying symptoms. But some of the foods would actually act as antidotes to reset her burners.

Andrea's immune system, her gatekeeper, had learned to react, via scent and taste, to almost everything in her daily environment! This can relate to an imbalance in the gut, but in Andrea's case, it was more likely that she was a sensitive sniffer, like the Celestial Seasonings taster, but she had never harnessed her gift.

I taught her the exercise "Adjusting the Flames," which stopped the lurching energies set off by the scents and tastes. By adjusting the flames whenever she got triggered, she could teach her body a new normal: balanced nonreactivity when exposed to most scents.

After about two months of adjusting her flames dozens of times a day, her system finally got the message, and her flames were able to hold steady. Her energies stopped reacting wildly to scents or tastes.

As a shortcut, she found she could use an antidote scent (such as vanilla) to counteract a budding reaction. When her moods started to teeter, she'd apply vanilla lip gloss, and consciously breathe it in, while visualizing each flame holding steady. Over time, the scent of vanilla alone would cause her flames to balance.

If you suspect you need something to use as an antidote, balancer, or scent healer, you can use natural substances (teas, herbs, spices, and scents from nature) and experiment with their effects on you. Like with other aspects of the language of energy, I encourage you to build up your own vocabulary initially, rather than working from someone's predefined system. I've found, for example, that while lavender is relaxing for some people (which is the property usually ascribed to it), it can make others paranoid.

The best way to develop this gift is through trial and error and some judicious self-testing to see what your body falls toward or away from. In this case, fall toward is the desired result, and fall away is an expression of aversion.

• • • EXERCISE: ADJUSTING THE FLAMES • • •

In Chinese medicine, there is an energy called Triple Warmer, which is made up of energy burners that can be found in the gut at the Dan Tien point (second chakra), at the solar plexus (third chakra), and at the high heart (fourth chakra). Each of these burners energizes the functions in the part of the body where they sit and guides hormonal communications. I have added a fourth burner — at the third eye — which I call the Triple Axis Control Room, since it's a meeting place for the master glands that control hormones: hypothalamus, pineal, and pituitary (see figure 8).

Working with these four burners can help you balance immune system reactivity, hormones, and how your body distributes energies.

One of the easiest ways to work with your burners is to adjust the flames, as you would adjust burners on a stove.

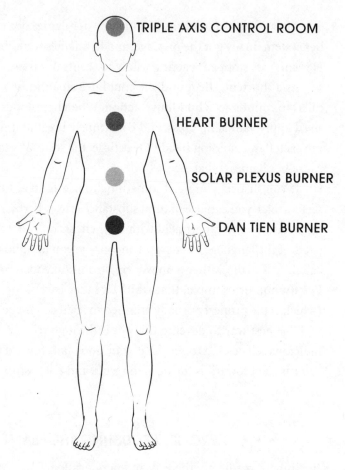

Figure 8. The four burners

1. Touch each burner with a three-finger notch (thumb, index, and middle fingers bunched together) and tune in to see whether it needs to be adjusted. Visualize it as a pilot light to see how strongly and brightly it is burning. You can also energy-test while holding the three-finger notch over the burner to see if the energy is flowing correctly (fall toward = correct flow; fall back = needs adjustment).

2. Imagine you have a dial in front of you, like on a gas stove. Use that dial to adjust the flame to where it needs to be, while keeping one hand on the burner in question. I encourage you

not to overthink it. Your hand will naturally adjust the flame if you allow it. (For normal circumstances, "medium" is probably the best setting.)

3.   Tune in once again to the flame and see if it is now where it needs to be. You can repeat the energy test if you want confirmation of your intuition.

• • • • • • •

INTENTION THAT HELPS GUIDE BEHAVIORS OF SUBTLE ENERGIES

'Twas brillig, and the slithy toves / Did gyre and gimble in the wabe: / All mimsy were the borogoves, / And the mome raths outgrabe.

— *Jabberwocky*, Lewis Carroll

Intention enhances communication. If I say random words, it might be entertaining, but if I say words, even nonsense words, and imbue them with meaning and the intention to communicate, they *do* communicate.

Intention is an important building block of the language of energy. Intention sets the scene in each action, interaction, and turn of the plot. Intention keys subtle energies to move in certain ways; it sets your energy field to both attract and reject events that will fulfill that intention.

It is important to understand the difference between *intention* and *control*. Self-help literature is rich in books touting methods to control your destiny, manifest your desires, and determine your health, wealth, and power in the world. In these systems, intention and control are nearly synonymous. But the implication is that you should decide what you want and get it. That is probably more linear than we are meant to grow. It doesn't leave room for your Wiser Self to guide the ship and your intuitive, creative self to evolve in unpredictable, nonlinear, and sometimes brilliant ways.

Life is full of plot we don't need to control. We cowrite the script, but we also jump into the drama just for the experience of it, to see what it feels like to take on that role, attempt that task, learn and evolve, and stretch our human or emotional muscles.

So when I say bring "intention" to your energy dialogue, I am using it in the sense of aiming, like we steer the ship, using whatever maps we can. The word stems from Latin and means "stretching, purpose." When we bring in intention, we are stretching to live fully and with purpose.

• • • PLAY WITH IT • • •

Lift your arm and make some kind of gesture in the air. Tune in to how that feels. Now make the same gesture, but imbue it with intention. How does that feel different?

Example: I make a circle in the air in front of me. It feels good, but I don't feel any particular effects from it. Then I make the same circle and an intention rises in me of erasing worry. It is as if I am wiping harsh words off a chalkboard and clearing it. When I do the gesture with this in mind, I feel the energy in my stomach and solar plexus area release some tension. I also notice I naturally exhale deeper and my shoulders and back relax a bit.

• • • • • •

Invitation, Invocation, and Inspiration

There are three specific types of intention we can use to help deepen communication and influence subtle energies:

- **Invitation:** We invite what we want: calling it in, opening the door.
- **Invocation:** We call on powers to witness, support, participate, and guide. When we call upon the subtle energies to bring needed resources, we are both asking for help from higher powers and trying to bring awareness and focus to what is needed.
- **Inspiration:** We aim to motivate, animate, rouse, stir, galvanize, and create. Energies move in response to inspiration

and often don't shift if we don't recognize what purpose they serve or what motivation they carry.

• • • PLAY WITH IT • • •

Experiment with all three types of intention. First, try invitation. Fill your hand with love, and then place your hand over your stomach and try to send it in. See what that feels like. Then invite your stomach to welcome that love in. Does that shift the feeling of transferring love? Too often we speak before the person (or energy) we are speaking to has located their desire to hear what we have to say. Once the receiver is ready to *invite* the communication or welcome it in, it flows more easily, they hear it better, and there is no need to push, force, or insist.

To practice invocation, place one hand somewhere on your body where you feel pain or restriction. Maybe it is a long-term pain or scar that you have given up on ever being able to fully heal. Holding that place, ask for loving intervention, for guidance on what resources might be helpful. Lovingly accept the pain exactly as it is now. Recognize ways it serves you. Then ask how you can be of service to it. Listen deeply. What comes up may not be words. You might get an image of drinking more water. Of gently tracing a specific shape over the area. Of shifting your attention to a whole other area of the body you would not logically connect to the pain. Trust this dialogue, and keep invoking help from your Wiser Self to understand, learn, and see what is needed. Let go of whatever end product your controlling mind wants to impose, and invoke powers greater than yourself to guide the dialogue over time.

To experiment with inspiration, tune in to an organ that is not functioning as well as you'd like (or to a sore knee or other challenged body part). Energy-test it by energy-localizing the area and using the Pendulum Self-Test. A weak test will validate that the energies there are challenged.

Imagine that body part is a sick child, and you work for the Make-A-Wish Foundation. Offer your imaginary sick child the chance to make a wish: What will give it meaning to keep healing? Imagine being the angel who fulfills that long-held desire. Then choose a souvenir or talisman from the imaginary outing or experience that you can use to reawaken a sense of motivation as you move forward. You can repeat the energy test to see if the energy of the pain has shifted, or just tune in to what feels different now.

• • • • • •

Intentions May Be Fulfilled in Mysterious Ways

Sister Maria Benedicta developed a cancerous growth on her foot. She was terrified of surgery, so she prayed and prayed for a miracle, asking God to remove the tumor. Nothing happened. She was bitterly disappointed in herself for asking God for such a favor and in God for not rewarding her piety with a miracle healing. Finally, she made her peace with it and let go, scheduling the surgery for the following week.

The night before the surgery, at around 5 AM, Sister Maria Benedicta was awakened by a blinding light streaming into her room. The light was pure and beautiful, and it streamed directly to her foot and the tumor. As she watched, the tumor shrank and shrank until it finally disappeared. She went back to sleep in a state of beatitude and gratitude for the miracle she had been granted.

The next morning, she went to see her doctor to let him know he could cancel the surgery. There was no sign of the tumor, and she could feel in her deepest self that it was gone. The doctor ran some tests and agreed; it was gone. She asked him: "Can you explain how this happened?" The doctor laughed and said: "I think that's your department, Sister, not mine!"

Ten years later, Sister Maria Benedicta came to see me about an elbow injury that wasn't healing. She was frustrated because it kept her from fulfilling her duties in the convent and in the school where she taught young children. She was exhausted, losing ground. She felt she was letting everyone down and was furious with herself that she couldn't let go and let God heal her once again. Surely she should have enough spiritual capital by now to bring on another miracle.

I asked her, "Do you need a miracle?"

"No," she said, "of course not! That miracle ten years ago was a turning point in my relationship with God."

"What do you need now?" I asked.

"I need the world to go away for three months so I can just stop using my arm and let it recover. But I can't! People are counting on me, and there is no one to take over my work."

"Well," I said, "I think your arm is asking you to listen to what you need. God appears to be answering your prayers with quite clear guidance: Take a break, get some rest, find help, and allow your body to accept the miracle of healing."

She looked at me for a moment with a mutinous expression, like a willful toddler, then she burst out laughing. "I'm ordering up a miracle so I can keep insisting on my path, and God is inviting me to take another path instead!"

"That's about it. That's your miracle: The guidance of everyday events is showing you what is needed. The situations that push you to really learn that lesson of 'thy will be done.'" She nodded brusquely, and I offered to show her some techniques to relieve the pain, while reminding her that the pain was her miracle message, and so the goal was to listen, learn, and follow the path it required in order to heal.

When you bring in intention, invitation, invocation, and inspiration, rather than trying to control energies, you find your way to miraculous healing in all its creative and sometimes crazy forms!

FIELD ENERGIES: ENVIRONMENTAL PLACEMENT AND ELEMENTS FROM NATURE

We have a kinship with chameleons: Our experiences are colored by our environments.

Environment shapes your experience and influences your subtle energies. Environments that drain you consistently can make you sick, as can overstimulating settings and situations that don't allow enough give-and-take. Conversely, wholesome environments will fuel you and support your well-being.

Think about all the environments you inhabit in your home, at work, and when you go out for events or to socialize. What is the balance of nature and concrete around you, of human-made and natural structures? What are the shapes, smells, sounds, and influences?

There is no one right balance of influences. Depending on how you are constructed, and what your energetic needs are, you might find comfort in a sidewalk to support you as you walk and a cubicle at work that limits distractions. On the other hand, it's good to be honest with yourself about how fully you inhabit each setting, and what those settings do to and for you. It is not necessary to study feng shui to investigate how environment affects you.

Example: I decide to do an inventory of how I move through my day, since my sleep has gotten restless, and I'm only sleeping about seven hours, though eight works better for my body. That morning, true confession, I look at my cell phone before even getting out of bed. A tempting headline pulls me into *Washington Post*–land, and my mind focuses like a laser on thoughts about politics. Ten minutes later, I can feel my breathing is shallow and my shoulders are tight. I open my shades and glance at the weeping willow outside. Oops, I've been tuning out this gift. So I stop and soak in the rays of sunshine and beautiful greens for a few minutes. I reanimate my breath, release my shoulders.

Then I head downstairs, where my partner has the radio on. The sound of the program, about the opioid epidemic, wraps me and becomes my world. Finally, I say: "Can we change the channel and put on music?"

That turns out to be the pattern for my whole day. Tracing my environments moment by moment, I notice that I am habitually ignoring what is overstimulating me or pulling me into worlds I don't want to inhabit, while I also ignore moments that could feed or balance me. I have become lazy about energetic placement lately — where I park my mind-body-spirit. When I don't notice my environments, I go to bed both unsatisfied with my day and overstimulated by it. In response to this inventory, personalized placement becomes a priority self-care practice for me: I need to notice, choose, and relate more consciously. As I do this consistently, my sleep again becomes deep and revitalizing.

As you learn to communicate with your energies, it is useful to explore and recognize how environment affects you.

First, we are creatures of nature. Most of us respond to some elements of nature. In chapter 9, I talk about working with the natural elements of water, wood (and plants), fire, earth, air, and metal. Each of these speaks directly to the subtle energies.

Second, we respond to sound, light, touch, stimulants, and all the building blocks I've detailed above. In that sense, it *matters* what you see around you, what the lights feel like, whether you are able to experience cycles of light and dark, of activity and rest, that fit your Earth Elemental rhythms. It matters if you go all day without touch, or if you guzzle stimulants or put chemical messengers into your body that mimic nutrition but don't actually provide it (think: diet soda, scented bathroom products, Muzak).

Third, we are a web of meaning. Therefore, the dramas you participate in greatly shape and influence how your energies flow and how well you can be. If you are working in a toxic workplace, where people are backstabbing and competing rather than collaborating, it will affect your body's biochemistry and ability to digest even if the toxic behaviors aren't aimed at you. If your internal chatter is a replication of the judges and critics from your past, that will affect your ability to be healthy and well. If you don't have work or activity that matters to you, it will drain your resources and call up loud objections from the body, mind, and spirit. If you do your work with a focus on pleasing others, so you can't find your own motivations within it, that also skews your web of meaning.

• • • PLAY WITH IT • • •

In moments when you feel polluted by environments that don't nourish you, try to segue out of that energy by getting yourself into nature: Spend a few minutes in a park, melding with the trees, grass, rocks, and water.

Try stepping into the shower and using your intention not just to clear the dirt of the day but also the environmental energies that set your subtle energies into a pattern you don't want to keep. Use your hands, singing or toning, gestures, and the water to clear and release what is not helpful and to invoke or call in a more positive color, sound, image, quality, and so on.

Even if you can't create a full immersive environment for yourself, you can gaze at a candle flame for a few minutes while just allowing your breath to deepen and your energies to open. You can do a set of energy medicine exercises designed to reset your system (see chapter 11). You can change your clothes to something more comfortable or comforting. You can hold a rock and feel its grounding solidity. You can spend a few minutes watering and talking to your plants. You can interact with a family pet.

The language of energy is the language of how you create a self, live a life, and relate to your own physicality, mental frameworks, inner landscapes, and spiritual urges. It is also the language of how you communicate and interact with others. It is richer, deeper, broader, and more multidimensional than spoken language. It is the language of healing because it is the way your mind, body, and spirit ultimately communicate and enact their truths.

• • • • • •

PRACTICE TIPS

- Pay attention to scents that knock you off-balance or bring you home to yourself. Similarly, experiment with tastes that can shift your mood. Find an antidote smell or taste that brings you home to yourself.
- For a period of several days, tune in to your four burners and adjust them, particularly when you notice your energy is low, congested, or otherwise out of balance. Whenever you react to a person, thought, or substance, try adjusting your flames to calm and neutralize the reaction.
- At the beginning of your day, practice inviting and invoking some quality, guidance, or inspirational perspective into your mind to guide your choices. Then periodically throughout the day, touch into that quality and reset your intention to welcome it into your energy field. At the end of the day, spend a few moments recognizing ways that your intention influenced you in a positive (or negative) way. Spend a few

moments thanking (and feeling grateful for) whatever guidance showed up.

- Whenever you have a symptom, illness, injury, or setback, ask yourself how that serves you. What are the gifts in it? Sometimes miracles, like gemstones, need to be liberated from the rock that encases them.
- Study yourself like a creature in nature. Explore which habitats enable you to thrive and which habitats cause you to lose track of your own pace, rhythm, agenda, or sense of purpose.

Chapter Seven

CONSTRUCTING A SELF

The *self* in self-healing is important. I've already said this in a number of ways: You don't just heal disease, like cancer or impetigo; you heal the self. It's not that the disease is irrelevant. It can give you clues about what is going awry or what is needed, often in a beautifully symbolic way. It can offer you an opportunity to stop forward motion in life to address what your body and spirit need and what they are asking the conscious mind to address.

But ultimately healing is rooted in honoring who you are by honoring:

- who your Talking Self is striving to be and become
- what your Earth Elemental Self is trying to embody
- what your Wiser Self is yearning to experience
- how well you coordinate your committee of body-mind-spirit

As a young child, you didn't just learn language; you learned to understand and sort your whole reality, while correlating language to it. On some level, you asked these questions:

- What was this *body* you were inhabiting, and what could you do with it?
- How could you get your *needs* met?
- How did this *world* around you work?
- What was your *experience* when you interacted with objects and events around you?
- Who was your evolving *self*?
- Who were your *people* and how were you connected to them?
- How could you get and give *love and joy*?
- How could you communicate to express your evolving *participation*?

These are actually great questions to revisit at junctions when your life gets stuck or your body's energies get bogged down!

When you were first learning language, it was embedded in your whole life. The language of energy is also embedded in your whole life. Self-healing using energy medicine is most profound when you can investigate how the construction of self is working for you across the spectrum of mind, body, and spirit.

Self-healing touches on all the ways energy is funded, moved, shaped, embodied, and released in all parts of your life and in all parts of your being. That is holistic in its largest and truest sense.

YOUR THREE SELVES

In everyday language, we talk about the *body*, *mind*, and *spirit* almost as separate things. But when I look at a person energetically, I see these three dimensions as interrelated within the spectrum of who they are. This doesn't take special psychic powers. Look in the mirror. It is not hard to see your body standing there, to recognize the personality and identity you are enacting in this life, and then to feel your spirit animating you and shining out your eyes.

In practical terms, it can be useful to understand the workings and communications of these three dimensions on their own terms. However, the best energy medicine addresses and works on all three levels.

My inner teachers introduced this concept over forty years ago.[6] They referred to the three primary densities within our consciousness as three interconnected selves:

- Your Earth Elemental Self, your body self, is a creature like all other creatures on the planet.
- Your Talking Self is the personality self who develops socially, engages in dramas and activities, plays various roles, and creates mental frameworks.
- Your Wiser Self, or Source Self, is the part of you that is rooted within the realm of spirit.

Although these three selves roughly correspond to body, mind, and spirit, I often find it gives me a better handle on what is happening energetically to use the terms Earth Elemental Self, Talking Self, and Wiser Self.

Each of these selves has its own focus, agenda, and sanctity to maintain. Yet they are also meant to work as a committee of three. Your Earth Elemental Self is designed to survive on a physical level, but it is also programmed to enact the dramas and embody the agendas of the Talking Self, who is busy creating a plot and characters and storyline in this life. And both Earth Elemental and Talking Selves are programmed to express, experience, and explore the energetic themes or truths chosen by the Wiser Self in creating this particular round of existence.

The Earth Elemental Self

The Earth Elemental Self is more than just my physical body. It is the part of me that is a creature, with creature instincts, like a dog or cat. And like a dog or cat, it will occasionally nip or growl at its owner if its sanctity is being violated in some way!

Earth Elemental has its own imperatives and agenda: first, to have an earth experience and survive as a creature; and second, to create an instrument for your mind and spirit to express themselves, explore, and create a life within this shared earth dimension. It is not just a vessel to inhabit; *it is an expression of your consciousness in physical form.*

Like all creatures, Earth Elemental Self has inbuilt instruments that allow it to be in alignment and communication with the natural world — with the earth itself and other living beings on the planet. It is part of an ecological balance of life-forms and can tell you many things about its own survival. In fact, it is designed to do just that: to give you constant messages and feedback about what your physical body needs in order to survive and thrive.

Its basic equipment includes the sense organs, brain, physical structures, and physical instincts. It is also designed to communicate with Talking Self and Wiser Self and other beings using telepathy, much as we are discovering dolphins, bees, and other animals do. This equipment, when it is working properly, helps you calibrate between your individual imperative to survive and grow and the imperatives of the more global collective consciousness.

Your Earth Elemental Self speaks to you through sensations, imagery, feeling states, telepathy, direct knowing, and sometimes even actions and events. Have you ever noticed yourself reaching unconsciously for a cookie, just moments after deciding to go on a diet? That is Earth Elemental Self weighing in on the question of whether reducing your stored resources fits with its agenda. Have you ever decided to work harder at the gym, only to pull a muscle a few moments later? Earth Elemental creates a situation in which you need what it needs: rest, to stop pushing forward on the physical level for a time, a different focus.

Earth Elemental's primary focus is in the present, the now. It is meant to be an anchor for you in the earth dimension, a self who determines ultimately how long you remain in body and with what quality of comfort, pleasure, and effectiveness.

However, your Earth Elemental Self is also programmed to embody and enact the agendas of the Talking Self and Wiser Self. Because of that, my body self might be regulating chemical communications and circulation related to digesting my dinner and sitting on a couch, and at the same time, it may be running chemicals and communicating frantically to protect me from the sinking of the *Titanic*, which I am reliving as I watch a movie and as my Talking Self identifies with the characters, plot, and atmosphere of that reality.

In many ways, our electronic, virtual culture asks more and more of

Earth Elemental Self. An important aspect of energy medicine is to help you evolve your ability to hold your own chemically and energetically in the face of multiple agendas.

Here are some simple energy medicine tools to help the rhythms of your Earth Elemental Self hold its own in the face of multiple Talking Self influences:

- Try slowly tapping your foot and breathing in an exaggeratedly slow rhythm, in counterpoint to the pace of whatever drama is playing out around you or on the screen while you are watching a show.
- Hold your hands flat over your stomach and heart, or heart chakra, while you are exposed to someone else's drama, reinforcing your body's sense of self.
- Hold a large earth stone (comfortable for your hand) and periodically tune in to its earth rhythms.
- When you are having "screen time," break visual contact with the screen periodically for the space of three deep breaths. (This is even more effective with your hands on your solar plexus and heart.)
- Do a *belly button–third eye Hook-Up*: Use your middle fingers and place one in your belly button and the other on your third eye. Pull gently upward with both fingers. Hold it until you take a deep breath.
- Sip water, slowly and deliberately, feeling the water in your mouth, and following its progress down your throat and into your stomach.

Talking Self

Talking Self is probably the *you* that you consider most fully your individual self. It is the set of identities that evolve in this lifetime; it's the mind that says, *I'm this kind of person, but not like that.* It sets up goals, frameworks, expectations, plans, projects, plotlines, and roles to create a life. It is most often associated with the mind, but it is more than just thought processes and beliefs. It is a dimension of your consciousness that your

Wiser Self comes into body to create, just as an actor takes on many roles within a long acting career.

The job of your Talking Self is to weave and embroider the web of meaning that is your life. You don't come into this life as a fully formed Talking Self. It evolves as you grow and experience your instrument and environments. But you do come in with predilections and gifts that help guide the choices you make. I think of it as being like an improvisational actor who has been given a few instructions: "Okay, you'll be female. You're going to be born in Omaha, in a household where people argue a lot. You're going to be strongly attracted to everything that flies, and you'll meet up with the following five actors at key moments to have some significant interactions."

These instructions are coded into the body-mind by your Wiser Self as a kind of warp onto which you can weave the woof of your life, with all its rich details and experiences. However, each self has free will to change both the warp and the woof. So sometimes you end up living many lifetimes in one!

Talking Self is designed to be the deciding self who steers the ship. It dances through time and space and different dimensions of reality, which we call *imagination*, but which is actually the larger territory our consciousness is able to span. One moment my Talking Self is feeling the keys as I type and the warmth of a blanket on my lap, and noticing all the signals from Earth Elemental Self, and the next moment she is in Maine, visiting a friend and imagining a conversation with her. One moment my Talking Self is an adult woman, more or less in the *now* of my life movie, and another moment she is back in childhood, or remembering past lives, or imagining herself as someone else altogether!

Talking Self stores dramas, goals, understandings, and experiences in your brain and physical memory, in body memory, in the chakras (which are like energetic storage units), and in the automated habits that get set up as we learn how to be a person in this life.

Wiser Self

Wiser Self is the part of you that feeds and fuels the work of your Earth Elemental Self and Talking Self with radiance, life force, and deeper purpose. Wiser Self is rooted in a dimension of reality that transcends the personal and the specifics of this life. If you believe in multiple lives, Wiser Self is the consciousness that contains *all* your lifetimes, all your expressions of self. If this life is a leaf, Wiser Self is the whole bush that gives life to that leaf and is in turn enlivened by that leaf.

It is Wiser Self that guides you, via your Earth Elemental Self, via the quiet voice within, and via signals, signs, events, and other symbolic means that illuminate the understanding of Talking Self. Wiser Self creates a larger plan for you, coded into the circuitry of body and mind. It radiates key purpose within you, when you can hear it, in alignment with your larger nature.

THREE AGENDAS

Each of your three selves carries its own agenda, and so wellness involves making space for each agenda to be fulfilled. Each self has its own sense of what is needed for survival:

- Your Earth Elemental Self needs to be heard, nourished, used, and inhabited respectfully.
- Your Talking Self needs to be able to create plans and projects that allow for its own fulfillment, while enabling your body's rhythms to thrive and aligning with your soul's truths.
- Your Wiser Self needs to be heard and to fuel practices that are in alignment with the purpose it has set and agreed to fund.

I know many traditions see the spiritual dimension as higher, or the mind as paramount, or even the body as the temple for spirit, with the mind as an interloper. But I believe all three are of equal importance in this earth experience we are living! Self-healing is most effective when it includes attention to all three dimensions.

Because our society often separates the physical from the mind and emotions and from the spiritual, it becomes your job as a self-healer to keep these three dimensions of self in mind as you address the challenges in your life.

Here is an incident of falling away from wellness that showed up on my radar while I was writing this book:

Day one: After a delicious breakfast of some organic turkey piled high with avocado, sprouts, and raw sauerkraut, I developed a sore, acid stomach. I drank something creamy, sedated my stomach meridian, and my discomfort faded as the day wore on.

Day two: I had another delicious serving of turkey piled with raw sauerkraut and sprouts. This time my stomach shouted louder, protesting with acid, gurgles, and cramping that progressed downward as the day wore on. I took some oil of oregano to kill bacteria and threw out the sauerkraut, which I energy-tested on a family member and decided was bad.

Day three: My stomach was too sore to handle my normal healthy breakfast. My Earth Elemental Self made it very clear what she wanted in order to feel better: half a gluten-free bun and some chocolate milkshake! Nothing else sounded palatable. Since I try to avoid sugar and heavy carbs, this got my attention. Earth Elemental was clearly trying to give me a message beyond telling me to throw out the sauerkraut.

So I stepped back to look at what each self was putting into the equation. The effects of the sauerkraut affair were that I could not concentrate to write, and I was grumpy. Also, the imbalance in my energies triggered my Earth Elemental Self's favorite *flag*: a mild migraine. Depending on where the migraine presses, I will get a variety of emotions that blessedly lift if I manage to clear it. Day three's migraine was pressing on my will-to-live button. A voice in my head kept saying, *I don't want to be here, I don't want to be alive.*

I could get into a whole analysis about whether this was a physical problem I was reacting to emotionally, or an emotional issue I was somatizing physically, or some kind of deep spiritual drama playing out. But the fact is, almost every illness or mishap reflects all three. Imbalance affects our entire spectrum of being. Addressing it is more effective when we recognize the participation of each self.

So I put my hands on my sore gut and my heart and tuned in. What did each of my selves have to say?

The Talking Self was saying: *It's not fair, I ate the perfect breakfast, and my body just reacted to it. What is wrong with this stupid body? Why does she have to be so sensitive? Maybe it's just bad sauerkraut and I didn't do anything wrong!*

My Earth Elemental Self was saying, through its symptoms: *Nope, not perfect. I didn't like that and you weren't listening. I want you to pay more attention to what I want and need today, now, not just follow another stupid old eating plan. It's not just bad sauerkraut. Don't you remember last week, when I objected to the organic spinach you were loading into your health shakes? I don't want to live with a Talking Self who listens to some health guru instead of me! Stop following intellectual theories and start listening better!*

And my Wiser Self was saying: *Your food plan is in conflict with your choice to learn deeper attunement, deeper understanding of the healing process, which is part of your soul's agenda and the topic of the book you are writing. You are being asked by your three selves to walk your talk.*

Bummer. Does this mean I always have to be perfectly attuned or my body will mutiny? No, but for a time, my Earth Elemental Self was clearly asking my Talking Self to align with my larger intention of attunement so my three selves could shift an old pattern.

I continue to use oil of oregano, probiotics, and acupressure in case my body needs help with a bacterium. But I also do some energy medicine to align my three selves, and I resolve to pay more attention to my body's input, listening to signals and energy-testing foods before I eat them. When I did that, it turned out my body wasn't really craving the chocolate milkshake (but it did want a banana protein shake), and it didn't really need the bun (it was fine with a healthier carb, but it definitely wanted a carb).

• • • EXERCISE: ALIGNING THE THREE SELVES • • •

There are physical access points to energy systems located all over the body. An excellent access point for communicating energetically with the Earth Elemental Self is the *sacrum*, the triangular bone at the base of the spine. An access point for the Talking Self is at the top of the spine, in the indent where the spine meets the skull (called the *power point* in Eden Energy Medicine). An access point for the Wiser Self is the *third eye*, about three-quarters of an inch above the space between your eyebrows.

Hold your sacrum with one palm (or bunched fingertips) and your power point with the other. Imagine a figure eight of energy traveling back and forth between your two hands. (If you can't physically do this, ask someone to help, use your imagination, or use a picture of yourself and send your energy to the points.)

Alternatively, you can imagine the hand on your sacrum is sending a spiral of energy traveling up to your power point, and the hand on the power point is sending another spiral of energy traveling down to the sacrum. Feel them interweaving like a double helix.

When you feel the figure eight or double helix settle into a good, smooth unified rhythm, shift your top hand from the power point to the third eye, linking Earth Elemental Self (sacrum) and Wiser Self (third eye). Allow this connection to figure-eight or spiral until it achieves a smooth rhythm.

Then shift your bottom hand from the sacrum to the power point, linking Talking Self (power point) with Wiser Self (third eye). Once again, allow a smooth figure eight or double helix to form between your two hands.

• • • • • •

A BRIEF INTRODUCTION TO THE GATEKEEPER

Built into every energy system of the body, into your nature, are two complementary mechanisms or forces:

- The radiance of your spirit that fuels and feeds you
- The gatekeeper that keeps you focused and safe

The radiance is your expansive force, and the gatekeeper is your limiting force. But they are both more complex and nuanced than that.

The job of the radiance is to bring in your spiritual feed: the streams of energy that fuel and animate you in this lifetime. In some ways it is like the drumbeat of your nature, giving you the rhythm that moves your song forward. Most of us have experienced moments when radiance steps up to supercharge a situation and accelerate our evolution. We often experience it as inspiration, an aha moment, a rise in passion, a gift from Divine Source, a moment of grace.

The job of your gatekeeper is to keep the gates of self, to keep you in this life. It is your physical, emotional, mental, and spiritual immune system. The gatekeeper is like a bouncer at a bar: It determines who can come in and who needs to stay out. It also breaks up fights and keeps the peace by ejecting elements it sees as dangerous or unruly.

Every cell of the body, and every energy system that makes you up, has both the radiance (the energetic feed) and the gatekeeper (the limiting, shaping factor). I see them as cosmic partners in a dance of fueling and shaping, expanding and limiting, animating and pruning the processes of our selves.

Wellness happens when your radiant feeds are flowing into your energy systems and your gatekeeper is regulating the maintenance of self. I will address the radiant feeds more fully in the next chapter, but it is crucial to first understand the role of your gatekeeper in constructing and maintaining a self.

All the body's immune processes and healing processes are gatekeeping processes. Inflammation, attack of cells or organisms, activation of tissue repair, and so on are all part of the gatekeeper's four mandates:

1. To maintain the sanctity of the self — keeping you safe and sound
2. To create identity — determining what is *me* and *not me* and repelling the *not me*
3. To regulate the distribution of energies — deciding where energies will be allocated, in alignment with safety and identity
4. To keep the habits — maintaining the energies' autopilot, so your body and mind can function without constant manual steering of the ship

This may all sound like an elaborate fairy tale to personify the processes of expansion and feed (radiance) and of limit and distribution (gatekeeper). But I have found that if we understand the gatekeeping and radiant dimensions of our being, and understand their workings as mechanisms within us, we have a better chance of becoming fluent in the language of energy embedded in all that we are.

The gatekeeper is like your home burglar alarm: It will go off when triggered, not necessarily recognizing whether you are a burglar or the homeowner! It is a mechanism that can be programmed, but because it has been programmed endlessly throughout this life (and others), you may find you are often running into gatekeeper reactions from when you were three, twelve, or twenty-seven. (For more on the importance of gate-keeping to well-being, see chapter 10.)

My inner teachers first described the gatekeeper as a corps of robots patrolling the energy field, programmed to react to certain configurations. For example, imagine you are three years old and your babysitter thinks it is a fun game to lift you, turn you upside down, and pretend she's going to drop you. She is laughing and swinging you wildly, and you are scream-ing with terror, thinking: *I'm gonna die.* In that moment, your gatekeeper triggers all kinds of self-protective behaviors and chemicals: adrenaline to power fight-or-flight, accelerated breathing to power kicking or scream-ing, and muscle shifts to make you go rigid or slack, depending on what your gatekeeper determines to be most effective.

Your mind programs a gatekeeper robot to recognize this danger in the future. The program may include aversion to this particular babysit-ter; a beating heart and a flood of adrenaline whenever someone with long dark hair in a ponytail like your babysitter reaches out to touch you; a sick feeling in your stomach when you smell the perfume she was wearing; and maybe even a sense of dread when your parents get ready to leave the house.

In the normal course of things, that gatekeeper robot gets erased when the babysitter realizes you didn't like it, brings you to earth softly, cuddles and consoles you while you release the tension in a fit of sobbing. She plays with you in a safe and calm manner for the rest of the evening. But all too often, those gatekeeper robots are not decommissioned. They remain in your field and get triggered whenever you see the same ponytail, smell the same perfume, or are lifted suddenly.

The gatekeeper is not in fact a corps of robots. It is a programmable feature of your body-mind that allows you to create and store *templates* of experiences, complete with instructions on how the autopilot should react or navigate. You've got lots of positive templates that allow you to do everyday tasks with ease and joy, and lots of alarm templates that guide you on how to keep safe when facing a similar situation.

When you recognize that your immune system is in fact part of your gatekeeper, and you have a physical, emotional, mental, and spiritual gatekeeper mechanism, it gives you wonderful tools for reprogramming your energy behaviors more consciously.

One of the best tools for erasing or at least calming gatekeeper reactivity and for reprogramming it is to invoke its cosmic partner: radiance. First of all, when there is energetic abundance, the gatekeeper relaxes and doesn't feel it needs to budget resources so tightly. Second, radiance soothes your gatekeeper, reminding it that in your essence, in your larger self, you are safe, even if you are experiencing threats in the storyline of your identity or body. Third, radiance offers a kind of energetic reboot, a return to the factory settings of your soul.

• • • EXERCISE: DIVINE HOOK-UP • • •

This very simple exercise is a good place to start to bring radiance to bear on a situation where the body needs more radiance. It invites the gatekeeper to chill and let more energies flow.

Using your index fingers, plug the left index finger into a source of radiance: the heart of the Divine (however you picture that), the heart of mother earth, or if you do not have a spiritual belief, perhaps into the heart of something you feel is sacred: truth, honor, kindness.

I recommend using the *action* of plugging in together with visualizing yourself plugging in, rather than just doing this exercise with your mind. The body generally responds more readily to enhanced gestures than to thoughts.

With your right hand or right index finger, you can now distribute the radiance to any part of your body or energy field that needs it.

Try a Divine Hook-Up between the heart of the Divine and your own heart area. If you are feeling a bit of tightness in your solar plexus, try plugging one finger into the heart of mother earth and distribute that energy into your stomach and solar plexus with your other hand.

You do not need to make the energy move with your mind. Instead, just open to having it move; let the Divine Hook-Up be like plugging into a wall socket. You don't plug your machine into the socket and then try to guide the electricity with your mind. You plug in and electricity flows. The same is true with a Divine Hook-Up.

Experiment with where in your body or field or even your life plot you can use a Divine Hook-Up to bring in resources.

Many spiritual traditions suggest a related but somewhat more mental practice: using gratitude or prayer or invoking a spirit to guide energies into the mind and energy field. Doing these in conjunction with a Divine Hook-Up can be powerful and lovely.

Finally, experiment to see whether plugging into Divine Source with the left or right hand is more effective for you.

• • • • • •

Finding Balance between Radiance and the Gatekeeper

Gatekeeping is necessary, not bad. However, a gatekeeper in reactivity or running amok is uncomfortable and can be found at the root of most illness. Sometimes you can also get flooded by too much radiance and lose your boundaries or definition. Then more gatekeeping is needed!

Radiance is meant to fuel you in measure with the gatekeeper in your creation of self. Occasionally, you can get flooded in a positive way and have moments of bliss, ecstasy, and expanded consciousness. But when your gatekeeper is disabled with certain drugs, or you ignore your limits for too long because you prefer radiant expansion to focused definition, then the gatekeeper can run amok when it comes back online, and mental or physical illness can result. I would describe someone having a manic episode as having too much radiance, not enough gatekeeper. Meanwhile, someone in a depressive episode has an overblown gatekeeper and not enough radiance coming in.

Barb's body was riddled with lymphoma that had metastasized and was no longer treatable with chemo. When we investigated her energies, her field was full of radiance, but her gatekeeper was both shut down and overreacting crazily. Her gatekeeper needed to be activated and supported, not calmed or deprogrammed. We used a number of techniques to get the cells to maintain their integrity, to reestablish their gatekeeping function again.[7]

This helped her blood cell counts improve considerably, and her family and friends were elated to think there was something she could do to reverse the metastases that didn't involve blasting her body with toxic medications. The techniques worked well for several weeks, but when I saw Barb again, she admitted she had stopped using the techniques and her blood cell counts were worsening. She said, "I realized that I want to be limitless. I want no barriers or gatekeeping. I realized that this cancer is taking me home to my soul. I don't want to leave my family, but I also don't want to force my body back into its box. As crazy as this may sound, I've come to see this cancer as my path home."

Healing is always about aligning body, mind, and soul, even if we are healing into death. Once Barb saw that she had a choice in what her gatekeeper could do, she chose to allow the radiance to rise and the gatekeeping to die down. She had a peaceful passing, without excessive pain, and she was able to convince her friends that she was not losing the battle, but instead achieving a passage her being chose to embrace.

CLEARING STORED TEMPLATES OF EXPERIENCE

Your three selves all store their learning in energetic templates. The gatekeeper is the keeper of your templates, your autopilot. To me, templates are like little computer programs the gatekeeper sets up in various storage places (chakras, body memory, the aura, and more) to help run the autopilot. If we don't clear unwanted templates, they can take over our physiology, thinking, and emotions when we least want them steering the ship.

Clearing templates can have far-reaching effects on your body, mind, emotions, and even life events and how people treat you.

Alexandra was facing a custody hearing for her children in court, but she suffered from a long-term issue with public speaking. When she tried . to speak up in public, she often either lost her voice or became totally scrambled energetically so she couldn't think straight.

We located the chakras where the templates for this aversion to public speaking were stored and used a variation on the exercise "Clearing Templates in the Chakras" (see below) to clear the templates. A few days later, she was in court, able to speak clearly and eloquently, and she was able to negotiate a fair agreement with her ex-husband and the courts on how to handle custody.

Another client, Cynthia, worked in a family candy business, but she had to leave because she became seriously reactive (experiencing anaphylactic shock) to the tree nuts used in the candies and the latex gloves she wore at work. This was a real crisis because the family business was close to her heart, and it provided her with enough income to cover her graduate school tuition. The reactivity appeared to be deeply entrenched; she had been working on it in therapy and with a naturopath for several years. But once she understood that she was dealing with energy templates, she was able to use the exercise below to clear her sensitivities completely within a single session.

Note: If the habit you are clearing involves physiological symptoms, make sure you work with your health care provider to safely expose yourself to the substance once again. Also, note that some templates are stored in multiple locations and can take more time to track and clear.

There are many new energy psychology techniques being developed to clear habits. For example, you may be familiar with meridian tapping (the Emotional Freedom Technique, or EFT). This method has you name a troublesome situation, such as a fear of heights. You are not asked to relive the situation, but just to name it well enough that your subconscious mind can pull up all the energetic files related to it. Then by tapping a series of acupoints while continuously invoking the situation, you train your meridians to stay balanced in the face of the issue. This effectively erases the old programming from the meridians and replaces it with a new template telling the autopilot to stay balanced in relation to heights.

Since a large percentage of your templates are stored in the chakras rather than the meridians, here is a quick and easy technique for clearing templates on a particular subject in a chakra.

• • • EXERCISE: CLEARING TEMPLATES IN THE CHAKRAS • • •

Bring to mind a habit or stuck memory you would like to clear. Name it and perhaps jot down some of the aspects of it.

Although it is possible to energy-test to figure out which chakras carry templates for your issue, in this simplified version, just clear the issue from each chakra in turn.

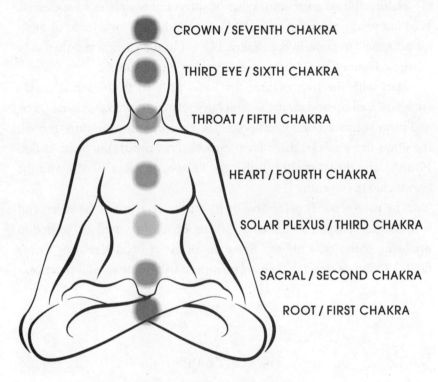

CROWN / SEVENTH CHAKRA

THIRD EYE / SIXTH CHAKRA

THROAT / FIFTH CHAKRA

HEART / FOURTH CHAKRA

SOLAR PLEXUS / THIRD CHAKRA

SACRAL / SECOND CHAKRA

ROOT / FIRST CHAKRA

Figure 9. The seven chakras

Place your hand over your root chakra. Call up all of the templates relating to the issue or habit you name, and then do a Divine Hook-Up (page 139) to bring in radiance. One index finger is plugged into the heart of the Divine. Your other index finger or palm is placed on the chakra you are clearing. Tune in to get a sense of when the radiance has cleared the templates for your issue from the root chakra. Often templates clear quickly. Although they may represent years of hard experience and deeply ingrained habits, the templates that store them are energy recordings and can be cleared or reset with radiance.

This is a little like selecting a set of files on your computer and moving them to another folder. You are not erasing memories or experiences, just rebalancing them energetically so they can serve as data but not instructions to the autopilot. What this means is that the next time you encounter a similar situation, you can choose new reactions, thoughts, emotions, and behaviors.

Nature abhors a vacuum. When you feel the templates have cleared, hold out your open palm to your Wiser Self and ask for a "seed of highest potential" to plant in the chakra. Place it in the chakra, and then do a "Cosmic Figure Eight" (see page 158) to help it take root.

Start with the root chakra (first) and proceed to the sacral chakra (second). Call up and clear the templates related to the same issue there, and plant your seed of highest potential. Then continue upward through the other five chakras: the solar plexus chakra (third), the heart chakra (fourth), the throat chakra (fifth), the third-eye chakra (sixth), and the crown chakra (seventh).

The gatekeeper is protective of its autopilot archives, however, and won't respond to requests such as: "Bring up all the templates related to my being chronically ill," or "Bring up all the templates relating to my faults." Template clearing is an art form; you will improve with practice.[8]

• • • • • •

PRACTICE TIPS

- If you hit a bump in the road — an illness, an accident, a breach in a relationship or job — use the list of questions at the start of this chapter (page 128) to assess how the bump is influencing all the dimensions of your being: your body, needs, world, experience of interactions, evolving self, people connected to you, ability to receive and give love and joy, and participation in life. What needs to be brought in to clear, open, and revitalize these parts of your web of meaning?

- In moments when you feel some resistance or conflict, tune in to each of your three selves to see what they want and to get them conversing. Often an energy logjam is due to differing agendas among the three dimensions of self.

- Cultivate a relationship with your body where you treat it like a beloved creature, like a dog, cat, or infant. Notice when you are snarling at your Earth Elemental Self or dismissing its needs as irrelevant. Learn what its go-to communications are that let you know it is feeling unheard. Play around with energetic ways to let it know it's been heard!

- If you find yourself spending a lot of time in Talking Self realms — watching screens, up in your head, texting and surfing the web — get in the habit of anchoring your Earth Elemental Self in the now by using the strategies listed under "The Earth Elemental Self" (page 131).

- The next time you find yourself reacting to something in a way that seems out of proportion to the event, try clearing the template that instructed your autopilot to react. You can either name it specifically or generically. If it's conflict with your brother, say, "I am calling up all the templates that caused me to [yell at my brother]." Or say, "I am calling up all the templates that make me feel [unsafe when I'm talking to my brother]." The more specific you can get, the more likely you are to clear the relevant templates.

Chapter Eight

ENERGETIC TRUTHS OF YOUR NATURE

The Radiant Feed

When someone is low on radiance, or has lost access to radiance, they can feel it. Others can feel it in them; there is something missing. In some people it shows up as low affect, a lack of vitality. In others, you might feel like there's nobody home when you look at them. I've even had clients who show up with their essential self trailing several feet behind them. Some people with low radiance seem a bit limp or low wattage. Others might appear rigid and tightly controlled, depending on how their gatekeepers react to the situation.

When you are inside the experience of having low radiance, you may find it extremely difficult to make decisions and choices. You might be short-tempered; experience depression, boredom, and blah; or get fixated on some distant goal you think will fix you, rather than reacting flexibly in each moment and letting yourself be guided from within.

When radiance is low, we almost always turn to outside authority to guide us, reverting to family rules and expectations, or buying self-help books and trying to follow someone else's prescription for success. Unfortunately, this doesn't work if you can't hear the inner truths that tell you what success looks like specifically for you.

Sometimes when radiance is lacking, we turn to self-medication, addictions, or obsessive love interests to fuel forward motion. One key to healing addiction is to rework your access to radiance and the relationship between your gatekeeper and radiant sourcing. The following exercise can help.

• • • EXERCISE: CLEAR FEAR, EASE EGO, • • • WELCOME WISER SELF

This exercise is designed to balance your gatekeeper and radiance. It can also help you open to hearing your intuition or guidance. It balances your ego in relation to perceiving energies. In other words, we hear guidance better if we aren't busy congratulating ourselves for how psychic we are or telling ourselves we have no intuition!

It first uses the exercise "Divine Hook-Up" (page 139) to calm the gatekeeper (clearing templates of fear) and to bring radiance to the heart and heart protector. Ego tends to relax when the heart is well fed. Then when fear and ego are balanced, you are invited to step into Wiser Self, integrating your three selves.

When doing the Divine Hook-Up, remember to use the *index* finger to plug into a source of Divine (or radiant) energy outside yourself, and with the other *index* finger (or full hand), bring that radiant energy to wherever it is needed in the body.

Clear Fear

Bring to mind your ability to use intuition, or whatever else your gatekeeper appears to be resisting. You don't have to list specifics; just tune in to what you are conscious of fearing or blocking.

Plug one index finger into Divine Source (the heart of the Divine or the heart of mother earth, for example), and the other index finger into your gamut point (in Chinese medicine, this is the third point on Triple Warmer meridian, TW3), which is on the back of the hand. The gamut point sits between the fourth and fifth fingers in the slight indent just below the knuckle (see figure 10).

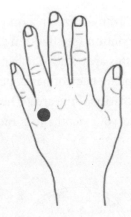

Figure 10. The gamut point

If you use your right index finger on the gamut point on your left hand, you can then extend that left hand and plug into Source with your left index finger.

Hold this Divine Hook-Up for a few minutes, until you feel a shift and/or release.

Doing the Divine Hook-Up on the gamut point goes into your gate-keeper's stored habits and helps to clear templates. It is especially good for fear or reactivity.

Ease Ego

This calms the part of the gatekeeper that guards the inner sanctity of your self (called the *yin gatekeeper*). It also helps to balance ego, which can block you from hearing your own truths.

To ease ego, do a Divine Hook-Up on the heart, placing your right hand flat on the heart, and plugging your left (receiving) index finger into Source. Hold for a few minutes until you feel the energies settle or you take a deep breath and relax.

Welcome Wiser Self

If you spend too much time in your everyday consciousness, you some-times lose touch with your Wiser Self. To welcome Wiser Self and open to

larger mind, first clear the "Ming-men" area on your spine — in back —
that sits opposite the belly button (see figure 11) in the vicinity of the L4
and L5 vertebrae. To clear this area, flip your hand back and forth on the
Ming-men several times (palm, back of hand, palm, back of hand). This
balances the plus-minus polarity of the area. The Ming-men is an energy
access point that leads into your depths to a radiant energy flow called
Penetrating Flow.

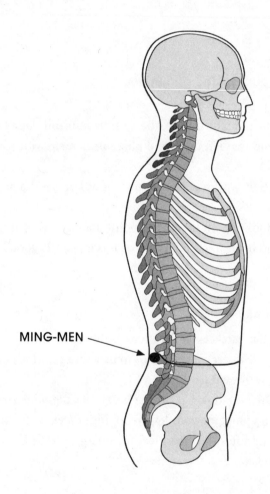

MING-MEN

Figure 11. The Ming-men area sits between the L4 and L5 vertebrae,
roughly opposite the belly button. *Ming-men* is a Chinese term that
translates as "gate of life," "gate of destiny," or "gate of power."

Then, imagine your Wiser Self standing directly behind you. Invite Wiser Self to step forward and connect its second chakra (between the belly button and pubis) with your Ming-men point, like a space shuttle docking on a space station. I imagine my Wiser Self as just a bit taller and larger than I am, so the two points align perfectly!

Once you are docked with your Wiser Self via the Ming-men, lean back into the support of your Wiser Self. Feel that energy feeding your back, your spine, and entering deep via Penetrating Flow. Then if you wish, as an additional connection, welcome Wiser Self to just step forward and *meld* with you, so you fully inhabit your Wiser Self and it fully envelops you. Feel how this bolsters and expands your senses. This is a lovely state in which to walk through your day!

● ● ● ● ● ●

SPIRIT FEEDS

Jim was a tall, very thin man in his early forties who slouched, as if trying to make himself take up as little space as possible. He seemed to apologize every other sentence. He described himself as stuck in life: emotionally, in his life path, and physically. He wasn't sick, but he almost never felt well.

Jim felt terrible about his life and himself because he had never figured out his life purpose. He was drifting aimlessly from task to task, able to get involved for a short time, but never sustaining any one job or purpose for more than a few weeks or months. He said: "I'm good at lots of things, but none of them really excite me long enough to pursue them and commit."

His major questions were: *What is my life purpose? What is my truest work? Why do I feel tired most of the time?*

His inner teachers' answer to his questions stunned him: "You are a tinkerer by nature. You are most fulfilled when you do a little of this, a little of that. Staying in one job, sustaining the same role in repetitive tasks over a long period of time (like working in a post office) would kill your spirit and exhaust you. That is why you keep shifting and changing. You are expressing your deepest nature. And you are tired all the time because you are fighting that impulse to shift and change; it drains you to resist your nature."

"Tinkerers," they explained, "are part of the tradition of nomads, itinerants, jacks-of-all-trades, people who move from place to place, act as generalists, contribute in dozens of small ways rather than in a single sustained way. Like bees cross-fertilize plants, tinkerers often cross-fertilize the settings they visit or work in. They are good at improvising tools and teaching little tricks to make things work better."

In this era of specialists and experts, Jim felt like a nothing and nobody. He came from an educated background, so his family was constantly encouraging him to find a passion and get a PhD. They even offered to pay for it. But rather than encouraging him, the offer deflated him, making him feel more apologetic, tired, and inadequate.

When Jim heard he was a tinkerer in his deepest nature, he sat up straight, and I could see his energies fluff up and start moving over the course of about a minute. He was practically glowing. And his energy level shifted from about a 3 to a 7 on a 1–10 scale.

"Do you mean, I don't need to get a PhD?" he asked.

"Not to fulfill your soul's purpose and nature," I replied. "But you do need to find ways to honor and embody that truth. In your culture, which financially awards experts, you might choose to become a professional jack-of-all-trades, an expert generalist. Or you might look for a setting in which your generalist nature will encounter an ever-changing set of tasks and challenges. Perhaps something like being a caretaker in a retreat center where you have opportunities to dabble in ideas and work on changing projects."

This story may sound more like career counseling than energy healing. But it isn't. Jim's energies were unfocused and blocked, and he was both tired all the time and ruining the health of his spine (which affects the nervous system) by expressing his self-denial physically.

By not understanding the nature of his particular spirit feeds, Jim was blocking his radiance.

We are each so very individual and different, even at our core, at the soul level. And if you are living a life or carrying a self-concept that is not expressive of your soul's truth, it will affect what your mind, body, and gatekeeper are willing to fund energetically. It will affect your physical health, your mental and emotional state, and your spiritual well-being.

If you are a mother in your nature and have no opportunities for caregiving, literally or figuratively, you will probably experience illness or dysfunction. If you are a navigator but have nothing to navigate, the frustration of that core truth will express itself in symptoms, which ironically then give you a healing journey to navigate. If you are a bridge builder but have no setting in which you can make linkages and build connections, that impulse can unbalance or overpower whatever identity you are trying to construct to please your family.

It is an important part of long-term, sustained healing to find metaphors that help you to understand your specific spirit feeds, the individualized energetic vibrations that make up your radiance.

Jim had signed on to a version of what a good, educated person does to contribute to society. It obscured his ability to recognize his own nature, which didn't fit that generic model. Because he didn't recognize his own nature, he saw the expressions of that nature as failure rather than as a valid way to be in the world. Finding a metaphor that encapsulated his individual nature allowed his energies to flow.

Finding Your Spirit Feeds

What I am calling *spirit feeds* or *radiant feeds* can be seen by people who see energies. I hear them. Just as when we filter a bright light through a prism and we see a rainbow of colors that are the components of that light, it is useful to view your radiance through a prism of everyday understanding and recognize the individual strands of meaning that feed you.

There are taxonomies available to help you learn more about your nature — systematic explanations of the different forms cosmic energies can take. Astrology, for example, offers a complex matrix of signs, positions in the heavens, and other factors to learn more about your gifts, nature, and challenges. The Enneagram is another system that categorizes types of people. A system called Life Colors correlates hues in a part of the auric field with individualized qualities and life challenges. All of these give you insight into your spiritual nature and what strands of meaning most feed you.

However, you can also discover your spiritual nature — and spirit feeds — by using your own terms to name your energetic truths. I believe that there are as many strands of meaning within radiance as there are ways within our language to encapsulate qualities and embody metaphoric roles or archetypes.

For example, here are some of my spirit feeds: I am a messenger, teacher, traveler, healer, singer, framer, storyteller, connector between heaven and earth, and visionary. Whenever I am doing a task that somehow embodies or uses these energies (one or several), I come alive. On the other hand, there are plenty of activities that don't allow me to use these energetic gifts and affinities. Doing those activities is possible, but it does not particularly feed or energize me.

You may notice I put the gifts in terms of roles, but this isn't necessary. You can also name actions or use phrases, like "I come alive when I weed the garden, sort things, clarify confusion, transform words into action," and so on.

My personal preference is to find ways to describe spirit feeds in slightly more metaphoric or archetypal terms. For instance, someone who loves to iron could call themselves an ironer, but a larger metaphoric role might be "smoother of the way." Someone who loves distilling words down to essential concepts could be called a distiller. But if that person loves other kinds of transformation, then an archetype such as "alchemist" might work better to describe their cosmic truth. Finding a metaphor or archetype that can encapsulate many expressions of your nature will encourage you to get creative in finding multiple ways to embody your deeper truth.

Here are some tips for figuring out your spirit feeds (or radiant feeds). You do not have to get this right on the first try. You can try a radiant feed on for size and see if it rings true; see if it opens your world or shuts you down. Over time, you will distill your list to the feeds that are most enduring and empowering for you.

1.   Make a list of all the qualities you feel are true of you or that you feel drawn to, such as roles, tasks, realms, favorite actions, affiliations, and so on. If you look around your house and see

five different collections, perhaps you are a "collector." If you love to try different flavors and ideas and even get to know different people, maybe you are a "sampler." If you feel alive when you are helping others, you have some kind of service feed. Maybe you are a facilitator, a paver of the way, a clearer of the path, a dispatcher, a caregiver.

2.   Although you may start with qualities, the goal is to find the larger energetic truth they point to. If you find you love to gossip, always wanting to stay on top of everyone's latest news, choose a name or phrase that captures the larger energetic truth; you are a networker, communicator, messenger, or storyteller. The point of finding the larger energetic truth is to support your use of the energy feed in positive forms. *Gossip* has a limiting implication. *Storyteller* or *networker* opens the world to other possibilities.

3.   Ask friends to do this exercise with you. How would they describe your qualities, gifts, and essence?

4.   Keep track of what excites you and what makes you feel alive. You don't need right answers. Start with a working model and keep refining it as you access your radiance.

5.   Although your ultimate goal is to find the positive energetic truths of your nature, sometimes negative qualities offer a doorway to recognizing spirit feeds in yourself or others. If people call you a complainer, are you perhaps in the larger sense a discerner or whistle-blower? If you have been kicked out of five apartments for being noisy, is there a gift of sound master or celebrator that needs a more positive outlet? If you have a friend who is always causing trouble or acting contrarian, it can really open your compassion to realize he probably has a "trickster" spirit feed.

6.   It is possible to use energy testing to help validate your hunches. But with energy testing, you are not asking your body to tell you true or false; you are trying to discover if your body's energies support a statement by funding it with energy. Using the Eden Energy Medicine Pendulum Self-Test

(page 94), say, "I am a [fill in the blank] at the cosmic level." If you sway strongly toward this truth, and away from other qualities, you can be pretty sure these others are not your spirit feeds. This can help validate your instincts. It is important to add the phrase "at the cosmic level," or something similar, to differentiate real-world roles from cosmic feeds.

Here are some possible spirit feeds to stimulate your imagination:

- Are you a planter of seeds, a harvester, a seamstress, a nurturer, a support person, a bridge builder, a seeder, a questioner, a challenger, a celebrator, a mourner, a visionary, a wanderer, an anchor, a pragmatist, a delver, a surface skimmer, a soarer, a walker between worlds?
- Are you a cosmic connector, an emissary, a grounder, a power transformer, a mapper, a wise grandmother, an unfolder, a communicator, a peacemaker, a mediator, a sacred clown, a sacred geometer, a cultural healer?
- Are you a protector of pure truth or of true justice, a ferryman, an awakener, a contemplative, a seeker, a troubadour, a poet, a builder, a stargazer, a connector of the dots, a keeper of the flames, a member of the psychic police, an adjudicator, a light bearer?

• • • EXERCISE: BRINGING IN YOUR SPIRIT FEEDS • • •

Find an image or photo that represents the essence of one of your radiant feeds and print it on a piece of paper, together with the name you have given that feed.

Stand (with bare feet if possible) on the paper and invite the energies of that stream to rise up through your feet and animate your energy circuits. Reach down and scoop up the energies, as if they are a wellspring of endless supply. Bring those scoops up to fill your energy field and distribute them to any part of your body.

Create a gesture that represents the truth of that radiant feed for you.

Use the gesture in conjunction with standing on the picture. After a few times, the gesture itself will evoke the radiant feed.

For example, after a long day of writing, I notice that my head starts to ache. My throat is tight, my gut is clenched, my well feels empty. So I print out a picture of a woman traveler, someone who is walking into a landscape glowing with light. I write "Traveler, Traveler, Traveler, Traveler" underneath. When I stand on this glyph that represents one of my radiant feeds, I immediately feel energy rising through my feet, like I'm a plant being watered. I scoop up the energy of this traveler and fill my field. Before I am done, I can feel that the tightness has released in head, gut, and throat.

To reinforce this effect, I create a gesture, rolling my hands outward from my center, like they are a wheel rolling forward. This releases even more tension from my head, gut, and throat.

The radiant feed continues to move in and flow where it needs to go; the well is refilling, renewing my flagging energies.

Save your representation of your spirit feed and use it consistently with your associated gesture over several days or even weeks. Make representations and gestures for each of your spirit feeds. Investigate whether you feel differences in the energy of each one. Investigate whether using the glyphs strengthens your ability to tune in to this feed and activate it when needed. Look for ways throughout your day to do activities that embody or activate your radiant feeds. Notice ways you naturally choose activities that are expressive of your spirit's sourcing.

• • • • • •

LIFE PURPOSE

The question I've been asked the most by clients looking for channeled guidance is: "What is my life purpose?" Without being flip, the answer to that is to fully experience this life! Of course, the Councils never stop there. They go on to explain the specific spirit feeds and themes and plot elements that frame that person's life. For one person, living this life might focus on primarily experiencing what the earth dimension has to offer.

For another there are some specific missions or intentions coded into their energy body.

These intentions are there as potential. As your three selves grow and evolve as a team, there are moment-by-moment choice points where you have free will to unfurl and grow, depending on the conditions of your life. While at the same time, like with plants, there are certain patterns of unfurling coded into the seed of your nature. This is not just true on the woo-woo level. Your physical body is coded with DNA that acts as a blueprint, but it also interacts with experience to determine what potentials get activated and expressed. At the same time, your cells are coded to learn from experience, which can then shift the DNA blueprint.[9]

I have found that we are usually born with the equipment that draws us to explore what the soul intended. We have inborn gifts and predilections, strengths and challenges that help us navigate the landscape our spirit set out to explore. Furthermore, we generally come through a doorway (a family, a geographical setting) or are drawn to dramas that bring those predilections and challenges to light. Self-healing involves both unpacking those gifts and strengths and addressing ways we might be blocking our ability to explore.

Use the exercise below to help integrate your full spectrum of being.

• • • EXERCISE: COSMIC FIGURE EIGHT • • •

The "cosmic figure eight" is a very large energy flow that travels between *Source, self,* and *world.* It carries energy from Divine Source into your body, out into the world of activities and shared energy exchange, returns energy to your body, and carries it back to Source, in constant renewal.

This large figure eight represents a pattern of energy movement that allows you to be fed by the inner wellsprings of your spirit, to use those springs to nourish and fuel your self, and then to further use that energy to power your work, play, relationships, and projects in the world. Energy and experience you take in from your interactions with the world further enrich and nourish you, and that feeds back to Source to enrich your soul or spirit.

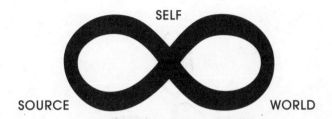

Figure 12. The Cosmic Figure Eight

It is an ongoing cyclic exchange. When the cosmic figure eight is flowing smoothly, you are more likely to thrive and be well. When you get stuck on one part of the figure eight — either too focused on the world, too preoccupied with your self/body, or too focused in spirit — the other two can languish and your mind or body will signal the imbalance via disturbances in their operations.

Trace the Cosmic Figure Eight

Trace the cosmic figure eight with your hands. This allows you to get information about where energy is moving smoothly and where it is getting bogged down. It also allows you to help move the energies along and smooth the flow.

Reach behind you with both hands to scoop up Source energy, bring it through your body, and out into the world in front of you, then cycle it back through your heart chakra to Source, and repeat the pattern several times. Pay attention to what the energy feels like as you do this.

If you are unable physically to do this motion, draw a stick figure on a piece of paper to represent yourself, then draw the figure eight on the piece of paper — so the eight goes from Source to stick figure to world and back — and use your imagination to feel the energies traveling through your body and field (see figure 13).

Personally, I find it works best for me to visualize Source as behind me and world ahead of me. But it might work better for you another way. Maybe Source is at the core of the earth, and world is all around you. Adjust the figure eight so it feels best for you.

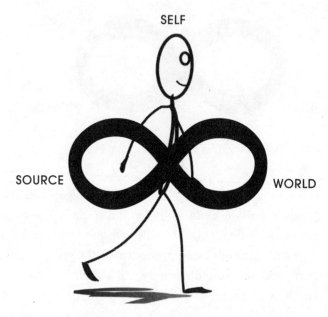

Figure 13. An alternative method for this exercise is to draw
a stick figure to trace the cosmic figure eight.

As you trace this, and any, figure eight, feel into the energy flow you are tracing. Notice where it is smooth and where it moves quicker or slower. Where is it most energized and where is the energy dull or even hard to feel? Where do you feel most at home? Most of us habitually park our attention somewhere along the figure eight.

After you have good information about the flow you are tracing, shift your intentions to reinforcing the figure eight, moving the flow, feeling it integrate the three realms it passes through, and everywhere on the figure eight in between.

By keeping your energies moving and humming throughout your spectrum of being, you are giving your system the resilience to heal, the energetic resources that support good health, and the rapport to communicate with you in whispers rather than shouts.

• • • • • •

PRACTICE TIPS

What does your construction and flow of self have to do with your everyday aches and pains, with that creeping crud that has settled in your throat, or with the chronic rashes that seem to show up without pattern? What does it have to do with MS or cancer? Most illness and injury arise as a result of gatekeeper reactivity and energy imbalance over time. When you work with gatekeeping, radiance, and your construction of self, you activate healing that is both specific and profound.

- Periodically during your day, take a sounding and ask: "What is the balance of gatekeeping and radiance in this moment?" If you find yourself mired in limits and rules, stressed about details, reacting and feeling prickly or threatened, use the exercise "Clear Fear, Ease Ego, Welcome Wiser Self" (page 148) to bring these cosmic partners back into balance. If you find you are so lost in radiance that you can't focus to take care of the needs of your Earth Elemental Self, return your attention to your breath, until you feel yourself land back in your body.

- Pay attention to what increases or enhances radiance for you. Radiance is different than excitement. Excitement might energize you, but it also drains you. Radiance gives you a sense of feeling energized, animated, alive, and fueled in a positive way, and it generally leaves you feeling fulfilled rather than drained. Radiance arises from a connection with your deeper self and purpose. What activities increase and support your radiance? Which activities drain your life force or unbalance your energies with excitement that makes you glow but leaves you feeling drained or diminished afterward?

- Keep a spirit-feed notebook to track insights about the particular nature and qualities of your spirit.

- Examine your life in relationship to your spirit feeds. If you have a nurturer spirit feed, do you have adequate opportunities to use that energy in your work and social life? Your health and well-being grow exponentially when you can explore and express your spirit-feed energies through the life you are living. If you are just doing work to earn money, and spending your time in ways that are recuperative, rather than celebrating your spirit's truth, your healing will rest in part on finding ways to honor your spiritual truth, even if it is just in your mind and imagination at first.

- Explore words that encapsulate your life purpose. What have your spirit, mind, and body chosen to explore and address in this lifetime? Sometimes purpose can be framed as a statement: "I came here to experience [fill in the blank]." Or, "My soul is trying to learn more about [fill in the blank]." For example: "I came here to experience my relationship with love and connection." Or, "My soul is trying to learn more about finding meaning in the face of obstructions." Sometimes our greatest challenges sit at the cutting edge of our life purpose.

Chapter Nine

NATURE PROVIDES THE GRAMMAR

It's Elemental

Although the word *grammar* might not excite you the way it does me, it essentially means the rules that govern a language. For the language of energy, nature provides the grammar. We are governed by the tides of light and dark; by the cycles of the sun, moon, and turning of the earth; and we are given meaning by the rules that influence how the elements of nature express themselves within us. In almost every system of energy healing, it is the principles of nature that guide your ability to heal.

The key to self-healing is rooted in your ability to communicate effectively with your elemental nature. Just as our number system has base 10 as its underlying organization, the language of energy has base *elements* at its core. We can't understand the language of energy, or of healing or wellness, without reference to this baseline nature.

Therefore, when you look at your energy body and how it speaks, you are looking at how nature plays out within you. Self-healing with energy medicine includes ways to work with the elements of nature in your mind-body and life.

You know how certain stories, especially ones from childhood, captivate your attention and stick in your mind? For me, true confession, it was the story of Heidi. In case that wasn't your obsession, here's what I remember: Heidi lived in the mountains of Switzerland with her beloved grandfather. They had a hut and goats and beautiful mountains and wild-flowers and lots of fresh milk. They lived an idyllic life.

Heidi's city-dwelling friend, Clara, on the other hand, was sickly. She was shuttled from doctor to doctor, overtreated and wrapped in wool, wheelchair-bound, pale, and weak. And most likely she was bored to tears. She lived in rooms with the curtains pulled shut to protect her from the sun's harsh light.

Somehow, Heidi, with Grandfather's help, convinced Clara's parents to allow her to visit them in their mountain home. Heidi was so excited to have Clara visit, and Clara was brave, and tremulous, and happy to sit on the porch and watch Heidi and the goats gambol.

But over time, something happened. Gradually, Clara began to take on color, fill out, and with Heidi's coaxing (and Grandfather's muscle), she allowed herself to be carried from her chair and placed in the grass, next to a tree, or to go on outings into the mountains, carried on Grand-father's strong back.

And when Clara's parents arrived at the end of the summer to pick up their daughter, they were met by a shocking sight: Clara, leaning only a lit-tle on Heidi's arm, walking step by step toward them. The girl who would never be able to walk had miraculously come alive.

I must have spent hours trying to parse the meaning of that story. It seemed to hold such profound truth, and I guess, given the path my life took, it was the first time I got to witness a miracle healing.

It has stuck in my mind all these years that a powerful path to healing is to visit Heidi and Grandfather — whatever that concept means for you. Wholesome environment, plentiful fresh healthy food, and appropriate, welcoming companions can heal you. Environment matters, the elements of nature matter, being welcomed to participate in a wholesome way of life matters.

Nate was, in his words, totally run down. Nate ate, slept, and worked his job every moment he could. He had been pushing to complete an im-portant three-year project, and when that was done, the backlog of un-attended tasks loomed over him. Finishing the project was a magnificent accomplishment; it left him in great shape financially. But the past three months, he'd been running on fumes.

Physically, he developed some very worrisome symptoms: periodic numbness in his limbs and weird tingling in his hands, even after a night's sleep. And he had a couple of episodes where it felt like his brain was just not plugged in and was faltering.

His doctor was in the process of testing him for MS, and he was terrified he might have developed it, since his cousin had the disorder.

Nate had heard that energy medicine can heal MS — Donna Eden, who popularized the term *energy medicine*, had used it to heal herself from severe MS. He decided to try it because he couldn't stand waiting around for test results and not doing anything.

When we checked Nate's energies, they were in a state of high alarm and reactivity. In fact, he could barely be energy-tested. His gatekeeper let itself answer one question, then it threw a whole array of baffles out to stop the dialogue. Nate's meridians reversed flow, he went into *porcupine reactivity* (for more on this, see "Porcupine Reset," page 201), and his heart protector locked down all his chakras, so he looked energetically like he was in a state of suspended animation.

It was not my job to confirm or rule out the diagnosis of MS. But it was clear I was dealing with a very freaked-out creature, not unlike the opossum who kept getting caught in our house when it came in through the cat door to chow down on kibbles. Any effort to calm Nate's gatekeeper seemed to just drive it further into reactivity.

Instead, I put him on the massage table and surrounded him with representatives of the five elements of Chinese medicine: water, wood, fire, earth, and metal. I asked him to shut his eyes and think about what color he longed for. He chose blue, so I covered him in a gauzy blue cloth and guided him on a visit to "Slow Time Island" (page 166), where a minute of our time becomes a full, lazy day.

Then I invited him to relax, enjoy the island, and left him to cook in the environment for about twenty more minutes. He fell asleep on the table.

When the process appeared to come to a stopping point, we gently checked in with his gatekeeper. Nate was no longer in porcupine reactivity, his chakras were flowing strongly, and he said he felt none of the MS symptoms.

We discussed ways he could sustain the feelings at home: setting up the five elements around his bed (with a crystal instead of a live flame for fire) and visiting Slow Time Island instead of drinking coffee at breaks. For about five days that worked well. On the sixth day, work took over his mind and body rhythms, and at the end of a ten-hour shift, he stumbled and nearly fell as he tried to walk to his car.

At his next session, we discussed the story of Heidi and Clara. "What landscape does your soul crave?" I asked. He had some trouble coming up with it. First he said: "Beach." But then he said, "No, that feels too hot and frantic. I think I'd like to be in the cool, green woods, maybe by myself, with no computers or phones. When I was a kid, my happiest memories were of exploring the woods behind our house."

I asked if he was willing to literally take himself to the woods somewhere for a weekend or longer. He said he was. It clearly wasn't working to just invoke balanced nature: He needed to live it. I got a call from him that night. He had booked himself into a ten-day silent meditation retreat at a forest monastery. He realized after he left my office that he wasn't just craving nature, but also people with calm souls. His workplace was such an adrenaline-driven environment. At the retreat center he'd chosen, there was no pressure to participate, they served healthy vegetarian food, and he would be able to pick and choose how much to be around people, while feeling his way into solitude.

Nate experienced a profound shift as a result of that retreat and took an extended leave from his job to explore how to rework his life and work. His MS-like symptoms completely receded over the next month, and his medical testing ruled out damaging plaque in his brain.

• • • MEDITATION: SLOW TIME ISLAND • • •

Have a friend read this for you or record it for a self-guided tour. Also feel free to adapt this meditation to the landscape your soul and body are craving.

Shut your eyes and imagine yourself on a tropical island. You are lying on the beach. The sun is warm, comfortable. The water is lapping on the shore. Light breezes play over you, keeping you at a steady temperature. It is a perfect day, with a sky of bright blue. You have the whole place to yourself, nowhere to be, nothing to accomplish. A cool drink waits on a tray beside you.

And imagine that this is not just any island. It is a place called Slow Time Island. Here, time moves much more slowly than in your everyday reality. As you spend a minute or two of your normal everyday time on this island, it is as if a whole day is slowly unfolding. Time moves so slowly that in seven minutes of your normal time, you can feel yourself taking a week's vacation on Slow Time Island.

Let yourself feel the week passing. Let your mind and body relax deeply with this vacation. Let your mind slowly untangle and sort through its confusions and your heart open gradually to this protective and utterly safe haven you have found. Let your breathing be guided by the lapping of the waves. Let the sounds of the surf be your lullaby.

As you open your eyes and return your awareness to your normal-time surroundings, remember how wonderful it felt to be on vacation. Remember, you have the power to visit Slow Time Island whenever you wish.

• • • • • •

CREATURES OF NATURE

We are creatures of nature — even those of us who are city dwellers and don't feature outdoor living as a big part of our lifestyle. Your body is composed of natural elements:

 the *water* that makes up over 50 percent of your body weight and supports the transport of nutrients

 the *wood* (plant power) that is your growth factor, coded into your hormones, your DNA seed material, and in the ways your body processes sunlight, derives nutrients from water, and requires rich environmental inputs in order to flourish the *fire* (heat and electricity) that fuels you via burning energy, regulates your body functions, and runs your nervous system and body's communications

 the *earth* materials your body is composed of that nourish and support its operation

 the *metal* in key elements that make up your cells and support functions like respiration, circulation, and reproduction

 the *air* that represents your vital exchange with your environment and fuels your blood and brain with oxygen

Like other living beings, you are designed to flow in cycles and patterns in attunement with the planet. Your well-being rests in part on being able to manage daily patterns of waking and sleep, action and rest, buildup and breakdown, and the ebb and flow of the tides in your body. Nature can be your teacher and your guide in this.

We also navigate our evolution via larger winds:

the **monthly patterns** of the moon that influence hormone communications

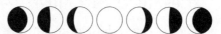

the **annual phases** of productivity and decline that align with the sun-tides and other gravitational pulls

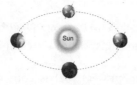

the **life cycles** that frame our social and lifestyle choices, as Earth Elemental Self evolves in concert with even longer seasons and cycles of growth and diminishment

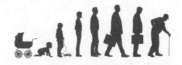

When Nate got sick, he wasn't just randomly struck by an MS-like illness. He had spent three long years ignoring his connections to nature, working against rather than with the rhythms that govern his Earth Elemental Self, and his gatekeeper was objecting by refusing to keep funding that way of being. The key to putting it right was to get him reconnected to the elements that could address his gatekeeper's concerns and heal him in a holistic way.

The elements of nature are *larger*, more potent, than we are:

 When I lie down on the earth and give myself over to her energies, she can realign and recalibrate my electromagnetic communications.

 When I lean against a tree and attune with it as a fellow consciousness, it can remind my Earth Elemental Self how to allow that vital flow between roots, trunk, and outreach. It can pull me into the present, with past and future in better relationship.

 When I immerse myself in the waters of the ocean or a lake, the flow of the water can reset my body's flows.

 When I sit by a campfire in the dark of an evening, I can let the interplay between dark and light, heat and cold, regulate my body's relationships to those dimensions: to the dark of the inner silence and the light of day, to the warmth of the heart and the deep cool night. I can let the dancing, sparking, shifting flames help release my overly controlled mind to travel in less linear ways.

 When I find myself on a mountain, with its metal-rock strength, I can let the conductivity of the metal and solidity of the earth negotiate with my soul and set me right.

 When I stand in a strong wind, I can let the flow of air cleanse me and clear my mind and field of all the stagnant energy that is clogging me.

The elements are bigger than me *and* they are within me. Their time frame is longer, and their rhythm modifies my rhythms and resets them to geological time.

It is effective medicine when you can get it. Often, we are so keyed to micromanage our healing, buying bottle after bottle of supplements to adjust our chemistry this way and that, we forget that we can also, like Clara, visit our wholesome relatives — the elemental forces — and let our bodies remember wellness.

ELEMENTAL EXPLORATIONS

Most healing traditions offer rich activities and sometimes detailed understandings of the elements and their interrelationships. For the purposes of understanding your body's language, I encourage you to build your own perceptions and connections to each element of nature and explore their interplay experientially as a baseline. Once you have done that, you can assess whether any of the traditional models works for you or whether you must, like many a good painter, mix your own colors to work with these aspects of your energy.

In suggesting larger encounters with nature, I don't want to imply that nature will always balance you. Too much time in water will overwhelm your water; getting too much sun or fire will burn you. Getting lost in the woods will befuddle you. When you use natural resources as a source of renewal, you don't want to abandon your own stewardship of body and mind or your own internal wisdom. However, when you find yourself seriously out of balance, getting into nature can be a great healing strategy.

In practical everyday terms, I may not always be able to arrange that. If I feel my health spiraling out of balance *now*, and I need to reset the rhythms of my elements, then I use ambassadors from each world.

Try the "Elemental Guidance" meditation below. Have a writing implement and some paper available to jot down your thoughts and perceptions. In this meditation I do not include a tangible representation of air as an element. Because we start with the breath, that is itself an encounter with the element of air.

• • • MEDITATION: ELEMENTAL GUIDANCE • • •

As preparation, gather a bowl of water (to represent water), a living plant (for wood), a lighted candle (fire), a stone (earth), and something metal, such as a bell or precious symbol wrought in metal. Put the elements to one side initially, and after you encounter each one during the meditation, you can place them as recommended around your body. You can do this exercise standing, sitting, or lying down.

To begin, spend several minutes just watching your breath come in and go out. Without trying to control it, notice where it moves comfortably and freely and where it gets stopped or truncated.

Notice not just the inhale and exhale, but the pauses at the end of each in-breath and out-breath. What happens to your body and mind in each part of this cycle?

Encounter the element of air in all its forms, as it enters the body, distributes, exits, and leaves you momentarily empty. Tune in to the reservoir of air around you, noting whether there are currents or it is still.

Now take into your hands your representative of water. Tune in to the water and interact with it if you wish: Sip it, touch it, rub some on your face. Then gaze into the water and ask: *What do I need from you today?*

No need to strain for answers or go into your thinking brain. Just listen and notice what images come to mind, what words pop into your head, what sensations or scenes appear. Commune with the water, and let it communicate with your Earth Elemental Self. Then, when you feel you have heard or taken in whatever guidance the water can give, place it behind you on the left-hand side (if you are sitting or standing) or just below your right foot (if you are lying down). The placement of each element around you will create a five-pointed star.

If you wish, take a few moments to jot down or record whatever came to you in your interactions with water.

Now take into your hands your representative of wood. Interact with it a bit: Feel the textures of the plant — its leaves, stalks, and where the roots connect to the stalk. Smell it and notice the interplay of colors. Feel into its life force, the green of it, the way it occupies space. Gaze at the living plant and ask: *What do I need from you today?*

As with water, let the life force in the living plant speak to you; let your mind open to images, sensations, and even thoughts or dramas. Feel the life cycle that is built into this living being, which sprouts from seed, grows toward sunlight, unfurls and flourishes, flowers, fruits, and then dies back to nourish its own continuation. When you have finished, place the plant on your left side if you are standing or sitting, and to your right side if you are lying down.

Take a few moments to jot down whatever communications you received from wood.

Now take into your hands your representative of fire. Tune in to the fire and interact with it a bit: Feel its heat, watch it moving and perhaps reacting to your breath; look at it through open, then partly closed, then closed eyes. Watch it affect the light in the room around you, noticing if it creates shadows. Then gaze at the fire and ask: *What do I need from you today?*

As with the first two elements, allow the fire to speak to your Earth Elemental Self in its own language. Listen in to the dialogue, and open to whatever guidance arises in relation to fire. Notice how it affects your physical and mental sensations. And when you have finished, place the representative of fire in front of you if you are standing or sitting, or if you are lying down, above your head on the bed or floor. (Be mindful, if you are using a flame, to place it safely.)

Take a few moments to jot down whatever communications you received from fire.

Now take into your hands your representative of earth. Tune in to the earth and interact with it a bit: Feel its texture and heft in your hand. Notice its temperature and how that temperature shifts the longer you hold it. Rub it on your skin, place it for a moment somewhere on your body where you feel drawn to place it. Gaze at the earth stone and ask: *What do I need from you today?*

Commune with your earth representative. Notice how it connects with you, how it communicates. What do you hear, feel, smell, see, and taste as you hold this representative of the earth? Do you feel any life force within it? Notice the pull between this earth representative you are holding and the earth beneath your feet. Pay attention to how it affects your sense of rhythm. Does it slow you down, speed you up, or shift your rhythm in any way?

When you have finished, place the representative of earth to the right of you if you are standing or sitting, or on your left-hand side if you are lying down.

Take a few moments to jot down whatever communications you received from earth.

Now take into your hands your representative of metal. Tune in to the metal and interact with it a bit: Tap it to see what sounds it makes. Feel its texture, and whatever texture might have been wrought upon it when it was shaped into an object. Notice whether it is still or whether there is resonance you can feel. Gaze at it, noticing ways it reflects light and shadow, and ask: *What do I need from you today?*

If it is a bell or gong, play it. If it is a piece of jewelry, place it where it wants to go on your body. If it is another form of metal, just hold it and allow it to speak to your Earth Elemental Self.

Notice how this element speaks to you. Are there thoughts or images, sensations, or perhaps just deep knowing? What is the voice of this element you are holding, and does it elicit echoes in any part of your being? When you hold it or wear it or listen to it, what happens to your body's communications and sensations?

And when you have finished, place the representative of metal behind and to the right of you if you are standing or sitting, or below your left foot if you are lying down.

Take a few moments to jot down whatever communications you received from metal.

Now, take a moment to notice that you are in a *field of energies* created by these five elements that surround you, and you are enlivened by the inhale and exhale of your breath. Let yourself bathe in that field for a time. Let the elements create their interrelationships around and through you. Let your own body's elements and rhythms submit to this field and be reminded of wholeness.

• • • • • •

ELEMENTAL BALANCE

The first time I encountered the five-pointed star as a representative of the elements, the Wiccan star, I immediately saw in my mind's eye the image superimposed on my body — the person as a star.

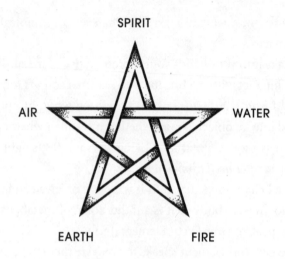

Figure 14. The Wiccan star

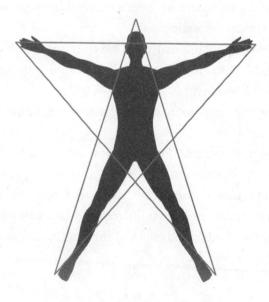

Figure 15. A person as a star

The five-pointed star is used ritually in earth religions and aboriginal cultures to call upon the four elements of earth, fire, air, and water, plus spirit (at the head). It struck me as a deeply powerful glyph, one of those universal ones that arise from the language of energy, like the heart shape, the spiral, and others that mimic the movements of energy.

In the image I saw, there were two built-in triangles. One triangle formed by the feet and head grounded me in earth and carried that grounded energy up to the heavens. The other triangle, grounded in my heart, was formed by my two outstretched arms reaching out to the world, with its point carrying that energy downward toward earth.

In Chinese medicine, the five-pointed star (figure 16) depicts the five elements — water, wood, fire, earth, and metal — which represent the movement and behaviors of all your subtle energies.

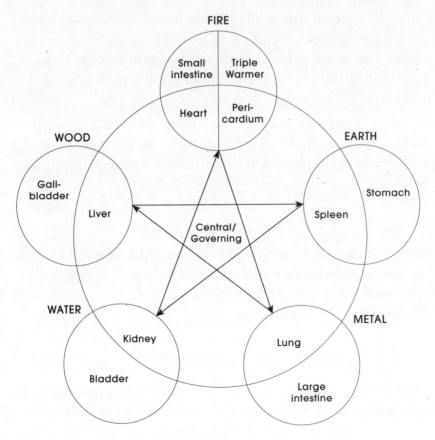

Figure 16. The Chinese five-element glyph

This more complex five-pointed star diagram shows the yin energy streams (meridians) that govern organs considered yin on the inside of the large circle, and the yang energy streams, governing organs considered yang, on the outside of the circle. Yin and yang are inward and outward energies that act like the in- and out-breaths to balance each element and serve as a pump to propel the five-element flow around the circle. That in-out pumping of yin and yang is air element, less visible but ever-present; the inhale and exhale that keep us in this life. Working with these elements and their interrelationships can influence your health on many levels.

There are several easy ways to work with elements fruitfully in self-healing:

1. Create a balanced field and place your mind-body energies within that field.
2. Use natural elements individually to rebalance specific energies that need support.
3. Use the five-pointed star glyph as a guide to reestablish overall balance and relationships among your elemental energies.

Note: If you want to pursue this further, many healing modalities, such as acupressure and Eden Energy Medicine, also address working with specific elements and their interrelationships to create more balance and wellness.

1. Create a Balanced Field

In the "Elemental Guidance" meditation (page 171), I describe how to create a star shape with the representatives of the five elements, which can serve as a balanced healing field of energy. This five-element bed (massage table) is the form I used with Nate.

• • • EXERCISE: FIVE-ELEMENT BED OR CHAIR • • •

Using representatives for each element, create a five-element star in the pattern represented by the Chinese five-element star (figure 16) around your chair or bed. For representative objects, you can use the following:

Water: Use a glass or bowl of water.

 Wood: Use a living plant or recently cut branch. Note that dead wood does not carry the same energy; if no living plant is available, a picture of a live tree is preferable to dead wood.

 Fire: Use a candle or clear crystal or light. Pay attention to fire hazards and don't leave candles burning unattended or near clothing!

 Earth: Use a stone or clay container.

 Metal: Use an object made of metal, such as a bell, spoon, or piece of jewelry. I don't recommend using coins, as these are too energetically murky.

If you are sitting inside the star, then put the fire in front of you, metal and water behind you, wood to the left, and earth to the right.

If you are lying down in the star, then put water at your right foot, metal at your left, wood at your right hand, earth at your left, and fire above your head.

Sit or lie within this field you have created for as long as you like. It can help deepen sleep, rebalance long-term imbalances, and strengthen the integration of subtle energies within you. It can also restore you if you feel energetically or emotionally drained.

• • • • • •

2. Use Natural Elements Individually

In addition to the whole field approach, you can use representatives of an individual element to rebalance it. I often carry an earth stone to help support and tonify my earth element, which easily gets befuddled. I frequently stop to commune with my house plants to help balance my committee of three selves, since plants, with their roots, trunk, and branches, span the three worlds.

You can use your understandings of each element as a gauge to get a profile of what your Earth Elemental Self is doing right now. Ask yourself the following types of questions:

  Water: On a scale from bone-dry to soaking wet, where am I right now, and where do I need to be?

 Wood: If I were a plant, what form of plant am I embodying, and what plant needs to show up energetically for the meeting I'm about to attend?

 Fire: On a scale of dark and cold to bright and hot, where am I and where would I like to be? Is my fire showing up as heat or light or both?

 Earth: Where am I in my earth cycles? Is it a time for planning the garden, preparing the earth, planting seeds, weeding and watering, culling and pruning, harvesting, restoring the soil, or resting fallow?

Metal: What style of metal is in me, and is it formed or raw? If I need more metal, what kind would I want to install? If I want to transform my metal, what kind of fire or light can I bring in to accomplish that? What form is appropriate for the metal resources I have within me at this time?

3. Use the Star as a Glyph to Rebalance Subtle Energies

This may seem like a strange phenomenon, but it works. You can use the five-pointed star as a guide or glyph to balance your subtle energies.[10] Place the image anywhere on the body where there is imbalance or dissonance, and trace the five-pointed star, then trace around the circle to reinforce it, following the patterns shown in figure 17.

The first pattern forms the bones of the star, the controls that keep its shape: Start at water, and trace from water to fire, fire to metal, metal to wood, wood to earth, and earth back to water.

Next, trace the circle clockwise, starting from water and going to wood to fire to earth to metal and back to water. That reinforces the flow of energies around the circle.

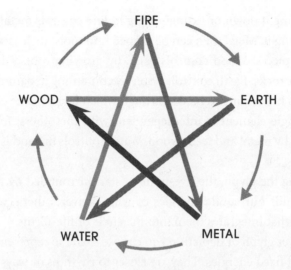

Figure 17. When tracing the Chinese five-element star, I suggest starting and ending with water. The lines that form the star represent the "control cycle"; the outer circle represents the "flow cycle."

THE INTERPLAY OF ELEMENTS WITHIN US

In the cultures that use this star image, the interrelationships between the elements of nature are encapsulated in the glyph and reflect ways to work with their interplay. The star shows an integrated way of understanding health and well-being. Tracing it acts as an energy unity, even if you aren't knowledgeable about the details of that system. But of course, learning the details can enrich your participation in the conversation.

For the purposes of this discussion, here is an example of the interplay of elements. Take another look at the Chinese medicine glyph (figure 16). It depicts the relationships of specific meridian flows, elements, and the yin-yang.

In the circular *flow cycle*: Water feeds wood. Wood burns to fuel fire. Fire burns wood into ash, creating earth. Earth minerals compress into metals, which are then born from the earth. Metal sweats when heated and cooled, creating condensation and water. Thus each element gives birth to the next; each rhythm activates the next.

With the five arms of the star, we see the *control cycle*: Water controls fire by cooling it down or extinguishing it. Fire controls metal by soften-ing or melting it. Metal then can be shaped into tools, such as an ax to cut wood into pieces. Wood controls earth by growing roots and breaking apart soil or rocks. Earth controls water by containing it, damming it, cre-ating basins to hold it and banks through which it can flow.

Any single element is interdependent with the others; for example, water is fed by metal and feeds wood. Water controls fire and is controlled by earth.

Drawing the glyph, the five-pointed star, surrounded by the flowing circle, reminds our subtle energies of what activates them, what drains them, and what integrates them into the circle of life-forms.

Whatever glyph or depiction you choose to use to represent elements, they are not fixed energies. They are closer to rhythms or ways for energy to move and behave and manifest.

• • • PLAY WITH IT • • •

Try placing the glyph on the floor and walking it as you would walk a lab-yrinth.[11] Walk the five-pointed *control cycle* (from water to fire to metal to wood to earth to water), and feel how it affects your sense of balance and control. Is some part of the star easier than others to travel?

Then walk the circular *flow cycle* (from water to wood to fire to earth to metal and back to water). Feel how walking each part of the star, then the circle, activates energies within you. Tune in to how doing this affects your overall flow.

Then try placing the glyph on any part of your body that needs help. Sometimes the simple act of tracing the star and circle over that body part will reestablish proper communications and energy flow in that area. It will promote and support healing. Fruitful places to try this are the fol-lowing: the Ming-men area of the spine (at the L4-L5 vertebrae), over the heart (the anatomical heart), over any chakra, on the palms of the hands or feet, on the whole belly/digestive area, over the face, over the base of the throat, over the power point at the base of the neck, and over any organ that is acting up.

• • • • • •

WORKING WITH CYCLES

Subtle energies, like all forces of nature, move in cycles; they are not a steady state. Recognizing cycles can guide your understanding of what is going on with your subtle energies.

The monthly cycle of the moon starts when it is dark, invisible, new. From there, it steadily waxes, light growing each night from a fragment to a quarter to a half to full at midmonth. And then it wanes over the second half of the month back to new.

This is how energy works in your body, your relationships, and your projects. It follows cycles. You may ask yourself: *Why can't I see clearly?* (a new moon condition), or *Why are things falling apart?* (a waning moon trait). The answer is because that is the nature of your energies — they start in darkness, build up and express, embody and take form, and then they decay and return to Source. If you know where you are in that cycle, you can learn to honor the new or waning times. If you don't, you may end up feeling you are failing at least half of the time!

The cycle of the day's activities follows the same pattern — the dawn of an idea on the darkened horizon grows into purpose and full engagement. Then as we tire, we sink down into reflection about where we've been and where we want to go next. At night we sleep, allowing the cells of our body to replenish and mend and our spirit to refresh its inspiration. If we only honor the activity but deny the importance of the downtime and rest, our bodies break down faster than they rebuild, and illness results.

Similarly, the wheel of the year has much to teach you about managing your energies over time. In the dark of winter, the ground is fallow and nothing can grow, and it is a good time to work on your tools. Then as the light returns with the turning of the season, and the ice and snow melt to soften and feed the soil, it is time to plan your plantings. As the light and warmth of the sun return, you can now plant seeds, which grow and evolve as the light waxes. Then the light and life force recede again. You cultivate your crops, the uncultivated plants go to seed, leaves fall to fertilize the soil, and the earth heads back to shorter days and rest.

For example, one day recently, I felt out of balance, overly hungry, upset, and disrupted, for no apparent reason. My first impulse was to ask: *What's wrong?* But I went inward to ask instead *What is going on?* and I got the image of a seed bursting into life, cracking the surface and breaking apart the soil. I could see that my behavior was not a failure, a hidden emotional issue, or a backslide, but instead it was an expression of where my energies were in their cycle. The disruption was perfectly in keeping with my larger cycle of growth in that moment.

It is so useful to work with models from nature. Think of the life cycle of plants and ask: *Where am I in my cycle of growth?* Consider the sun and moon and ask: *Where am I in the cycle of light and dark?* Or reflect on the wheel of the year and consider what season you are in and what that season is asking of you.

If we don't understand how nature moves through us, how cycles spiral us deeply into our experience, then we cannot effectively navigate the winds of change that blow through our lives and projects and relationships. We cannot understand the empowerment available to us as a gift of our human, earthbound nature.

Revisit the exercise "Shifting Cycles" (page 103) as you explore how cycles influence your efforts to thrive.

• • • PLAY WITH IT • • •

You do not need to study Chinese medicine to develop a personalized core vocabulary to perceive how nature is playing through you. Take what you know about each element and see how that is showing up in you.

Brainstorm with a group of friends about what forms each of the elements can take. For example, earth can be soil, sand, stone, rock, dirt, dust, and so on. It can be rich and fertile or arid and only able to support desert plants. Have each person jot down what their water, wood, fire, earth, metal, and air are like when they are balanced and out of balance.

For example, I tried this recently, and here's what I came up with:

My water is a burbling brook, but when I am out of balance, it is an algae-choked pond.
My wood is a weeping willow — lots of updraft, but some droopy downdraft as well. When it is out of balance, I'm a willow switch trying to clear a path in front of me.

My fire is a dancing, sometimes crackling campfire. But some-times it is more like the light of a lighthouse, illuminating the darkness. When it is out of balance, I burn too hot and too fast and the light can be blinding.

My earth is like rich loam (not stone), and when I am out of bal-ance, it moves like the earth moves in front of a bulldozer.

My metal is a scaffold, strong enough to hold up workers, but not strong enough to hold up a building. When it is out of bal-ance, I'm braces — too much metal, not enough teeth.

My air is an eddy, swirling and swooping, then dying down and picking up again. When it is out of balance, my air is an insis-tent wind, a little too pushy, or it is a doldrum.

• • • • • •

PRACTICE TIPS

Working with elements is a way to use the language of energy to assess the energetics of your body, your storyline, your choices, and your actions.

- Explore your personal relationship to each element: water, wood (or plant energy), fire, earth, metal, and air. How does each of these affect you? Which console and calm you, and which animate and move you?
- Next time you are feeling off-kilter, arrange to spend some time in a natural setting, and observe how you feel before, during, and after.
- Do an honest assessment of the role nature and the natu-ral world play in your life. How attuned are you to how the movements of the sun, the moon, and cycles affect you per-sonally? Can you look back at times in your life when you felt in sync with nature?
- Energy-localize places on your body where you feel distur-bance or imbalance (or pain or underperformance), and energy-test them. If they test weak, experiment with tracing

the five-pointed star glyph on that area. Trace the star (control cycle), then the circle (flow cycle), with intention and pay attention to how it feels. Does anything shift in your sensations, or if you post-test using an energy test?

• Whenever you need help to balance your subtle energies, or want to balance your mind and emotions, use a "Five-Element Bed or Chair" (page 176) for twenty to thirty minutes. See what shifts in your mind-body communications.

Chapter Ten

HEALING CONVERSATIONS

Energy Dialogue

As a young child, as you grew, your understanding of language broadened and deepened, and your ability to communicate grew exponentially. You moved from expressing ideas in two- and three-word sentences to learning how to link ideas, to generalize, and to express more complex relationships.

You moved from talking about and relating only what was happening for you to being able to actually *converse*. You moved from language that expressed direct needs and desires to a more nuanced ability to *participate*. You became able to think about and talk about experience, shared culture, and your growing understanding of the world.

This and the next chapter explore healing conversations — what it means to converse with more complexity and participate in the language of energy.

HEALING APPROACH

When I was growing up, our family pet was a rotund beagle mutt named Teeny. She had long droopy ears, soulful eyes, and a belly that nearly dragged on the ground. She woke up each day clearly happy to be a dog.

We were the same age, and in many ways she was one of my first teachers of energy healing. No matter what was ailing me, I could climb into the dirty clothes cupboard where Teeny liked to nap, cuddle up, and find relief. I would wrap myself around her, align my rhythms with her contented slumber, and feel my inner landscape shift and reorganize in response.

Teeny was a great communicator and was also great at getting love and teaching love. So here's one thing I learned: If I scratched Teeny's butt, it would make her feel good and get her tail wagging. It was quick and easy. But I would find myself with her unlovely butt in my face. On the other hand, if I caressed her ears and spoke to her, her tail would still wag to beat the band, but we would be face to face, exchanging soulful glances and basking in the love that flowed between us.

For some reason, that's what comes to my mind when I think about how to approach self-healing. Do I want to focus in on the tail area (the disease, the symptoms, the pain) and have the equivalent of a butt in my face? Or do I want to turn my attention to the front of the dog (supporting energies to move the way they are designed to move), have a face-to-face lovefest with my being, and send that energetic exchange cascading through my being to get my tail wagging? It is not an either/or proposition, of course. There are many ways to love up a dog and even more ways to enter into healing dialogue with all parts of yourself.

One of the principles of energy is that whatever we focus on gets energized. So if my focus is all on my illness, what is wrong, and what is going on with the chemistry and symptoms and biodynamics, then ultimately illness is what I am calling in. If we plant cauliflower seeds in the garden, cauliflower — and some weeds — will show up. That's why an important part of healing any disease is the willingness to plant and cultivate well-being, to call in the energies you want to embody.

Being well is not the same thing as having perfect health. Too often in our culture, cultivating wellness gets translated into hyper-vigilant perfectionism: I have to eat the perfect diet (and read all the experts arguing over what that would look like). I have to exercise to get fit and lean (and read the science of exercise so I know precisely what to do when). I have to meditate and do yoga, clear my psyche using therapy or tapping, clean up all of my relationships, and preferably find my soul mate, who will share all this self-improvement activity.

In themselves, these are not necessarily bad. But if the energy motivating my search for wellness is physical/energetic perfectionism, or it is rooted in following the rules and path someone else has laid out, irrespective of what my own being is trying to communicate, it can bypass my ability to find out what wellness and well-being look like for me.

Energy dialogue can lead to a more personalized, guided form of wellness: one that is in keeping with your elemental nature; that includes trial and error; that may be messy or elegant; and that will include occasional illness or unlovely symptoms and social-emotional experiments that don't work out precisely how you planned.

Energy dialogue can guide you along the path to wellness that aligns with your specific, spectacular soul. In the process, symptoms might dissipate quickly and even miraculously, or they might keep showing up to flag that your system still needs loving attention.

This kind of wellness involves finding an inner sense of rightness, of being on your path, of being truly alive and human, of *participating* in your own life. I believe it is a more enduring form of wellness than is represented by that glowing superhuman person selling you health products and claiming that they can show you the secret of how to be healthy, successful, gorgeous, and happy like them.

A QUICK REVIEW OF ENERGY DIALOGUE

Energy dialogue involves learning to communicate in a vital exchange with your own energetic nature, *using language your energies can understand.*

I tend to favor using vocabulary that is natural, that communicates with and via energy: touch, gestures, movements, imagery, sound, rhythm, and also everyday activities that can serve as "lifestyle medicine" (cleaning dirty dishes, organizing my shoes, clearing my schedule to create unstructured time). Sometimes I use something from nature to amplify my communications: a green leaf from a tree, an earth stone or crystal, a magnet, or other elemental ambassadors.

My personal vocabulary has expanded over the years to include the equivalent of idioms and phrases: energy exercises and techniques I've invented, as well as ones I've learned from other modalities. The exercises and techniques in chapters 10 and 11 are designed to broaden and deepen your ability to converse.

Your vocabulary might include tools or practices you gathered from healing and spiritual traditions like yoga and even from other realms — like the arts, philosophy, gaming, building, gardening, sports, and so on — that allow you to tune in to and interact with your web of meaning.

There are energy vocabulary tools that I don't tend to use, such as machines calibrated to pulse certain vibrations, magnet-embedded mattresses, and instruments designed to read subtle energies. Technology that can measure or influence your energies isn't bad, as long as it isn't used in place of actual perception and communication. But a machine can't have the same give-and-take, the same out-of-the-box thinking, or the same lovefest with my energies that I can have with natural tools. Therefore, trying to dialogue using an instrument becomes more about assessment and treatment — not allowing the full bandwidth of information to flow.

Just as words gain meaning from sentence structure and context, energy dialogue can deepen when we understand that the language of energy has syntax, arrangements of how subtle energies behave. When you hear people mention chakras, auras, meridians, and grid, they are referring to some of the ways subtle energy forms patterns of behavior that have been mapped in various traditions of healing.[12] In the six healing conversations in chapters 10 and 11, I introduce another kind of useful energy syntax, one organized around components of wellness, such as gatekeeping, grounding, rooting and anchoring, inner coherence, energetic exchange with others, energy flow, and radiance.

Finally, energy dialogue happens in the context of constructing a self, constructing a life. Your life and identity guide how energies are called in, circulate, and communicate with others. One person who believes she is good at math gets energized when she encounters a math problem. Another, believing he's not a math person, might feel exhausted and drained when confronted with a math problem. In both situations the energy flow is guided by who people believe themselves to be.

The whole point of language is to communicate, not just to say words or even to form sentences and paragraphs. When we learn energy medicine that addresses subtle energies in the context of constructing our web of meaning, we are more capable of participating in and contributing to the conversation.

SIX HEALING CONVERSATIONS

Noreen showed up in my office with a four-page typed list of symptoms and concerns. She had a great, somewhat self-effacing sense of humor and started our session by saying: "I have to warn you, I'm a train wreck!" Ironically, Noreen didn't strike me as a train wreck. She cracked jokes and had a strong intellect and a strong will to keep moving forward, which helped her to put brackets on the illness and try to live despite the pain and disruptions.

I must say, her list was impressive. She had several diagnoses of auto-immune disease (irritable bowel syndrome, lupus), multiple sensitivities and allergies, and a history of episodes that had been severe enough to land her in the hospital. Pneumonia was the most recent and involved not only a weeklong hospital stay on IV antibiotics, but about three months on the couch trying to recover her strength. Noreen had also undergone multiple surgeries over the years as a result of a knee injury in her teens.

She was a good example of someone who had spent so much time addressing illnesses and physical dysfunction, and the feelings arising from them, that she barely had time to think about what kind of life or wellness she wanted to create. When I asked her what her image of being well looked like, she threw the list in the wastebasket with a dramatic flourish. "This would all be gone," she said.

Most of us who have experienced chronic issues can relate to Noreen. When I had daily migraines, my vision of wellness started with "no headaches." It was a nightmarish broken record to keep repeating the migraine dance, day after day. But during that time, I never considered whether I could just accept myself as a whole person whose body was using migraines to flag what it needed. Migraines were evidence of my brokenness, the dysfunction of my metabolism, my failure to adequately cope with stress. For fifteen long years I was stuck on that hamster wheel of self-rejection and chronic pain.

Energy dialogue enabled me to shift the conversation and get off the hamster wheel. It does not require that you know precisely what is wrong or what to do about it. You just need to show up, listen, learn, and begin to support your body, mind, and spirit on their own terms.

First, I began doing a daily energy routine that supported my energies at the core, by helping them to move and connect.[13] By doing this, I was no longer focused on fixing what was wrong or treating symptoms. Instead, I was supporting and reinforcing my energies to move the way they needed to move.

Then, as I experienced more moments of flow and balance, the guidance that I found so easy to produce for others was clearer and available to me. There was space in my mind to entertain other options. I stopped obsessively planting the question "What's wrong?" in my garden, and instead I planted the question: "What can I do for you in this moment?" And the new crops gave my body new kinds of nourishment.

This was the approach Noreen learned to take: She put aside her list of symptoms and instead focused on building her core. Over time, each health challenge either dissipated or became a guide for Noreen to what was needed in order for her to shift her map of expression. Over the course of a year, Noreen's gatekeeper learned to trust her, and she learned to trust herself. Through that process, the autoimmune disorders cleared, allowing her body to turn its attention to healing the damaged tissues from her multiple surgeries.

In the six healing conversations that follow, I offer a set of specific energy medicine exercises, presented in the context of the energy issues they help you to address: gatekeeping (creating identity and boundaries); grounding; inner connection and coherence; exchange between self and world; resetting the body's energy flows; and bringing in radiance to fuel your purpose.

These are not the only fruitful conversations you can have. However, taken together and used as a daily energy routine, they greatly help to strengthen your energetic core.

Each exercise can be used with three distinct intentions:

1. **Assess**: Tune in to and discover how your energies are doing.
2. **Rebalance**: Reorganize, reinforce, and reanimate your energies.

3. **Invoke**: Call in what needs to be brought into your web of meaning to enrich your experience.

For example, if you were doing the exercise "Cosmic Figure Eight" (page 158), and tracing the figure eight that runs between Source, self, and world, you would simply do so as described in the instructions. However, as you trace, you can initially tune in and assess the energy you are encountering. Then, as you continue, you can shift your focus to rebalance the energies and, finally, to set an intention and invoke what is needed.

Assess

As you do an energy exercise, tune in and assess what you feel in your body and how it affects your mood and mind. This gives you a chance to get information about how that energy stream is moving in your life. As you do any exercise, feel into it. If you were doing "Cosmic Figure Eight," for example, here are some questions you might ask:

- At what pace are you tracing the figure eight, and does that feel like the right pace? What happens if you go slower or faster?
- Which parts of the eight are easy to trace, and where do you feel resistance, or wobbles, or something affecting your tracing?
- Are sensations arising in your hands, thoughts, or feelings as you draw the eight?
- Are you able to stay attuned to the energy as you trace the eight, or does your attention wander? Where on the eight do you lose your concentration, or feel it quickening?

Exploring these dimensions will give you information about what is needed. If you tune out each time you get to the "Source" position, maybe you need more attention to spirit. Similarly, if your hands move smoothly in the "world" position, perhaps that is where you have invested the most attention.

Note: You can use any energy medicine exercise as a way to assess and address the energy of a particular situation you are struggling with. First, do the exercise with a neutral mind, just letting the energies show you what is true now. Then, repeat the exercise, focusing on the particular situation you want to affect. For example, if you have a disagreement with a loved one that leaves you feeling upset, first do the "Cosmic Figure Eight" exercise normally, to balance the energies. Then bring the disagreement to mind and repeat the exercise. This will allow you to assess, rebalance, and invoke enhancements to shift your energetic relationship to the loved one.

Rebalance

Energy medicine exercises enable you to reorganize, reinforce, and re-animate energies that need support. Well-designed energy medicine exercises communicate with and reinforce your energies on many levels, rather than just fixing a flipped energy pattern or getting a flow going. If you pay attention to what you are doing, tuning in to the energies and the purpose for doing it, you will get even more benefit.

Adapt how you do an exercise to your present moment. Today, you might need a very slow and consoling movement, and next time, a more vigorous approach. Like with any conversation, adjust your contributions to what the energy is expressing. You will soon learn the art of supporting and reinforcing subtle energies in ways that bolster their ability to function.

Invoke

Beyond assessing your energies and promoting rebalance, you can also invoke help, qualities, and radiance you'd like to invite into the mix. In the "Cosmic Figure Eight" exercise, you might get a sense as you trace the figure eight that your energies are sluggish. Not stuck, but not energized. Fill your hands with love, bring in a color or an inspirational quality (like grace), and continue tracing the figure eight while inviting new energies into the flow. This is a wonderful way to call in reinforcements to enhance your subtle energies.

HOW ATTENTION TO YOUR ILLNESS AND PAIN CAN HELP

The goal of energy dialogue is to shift the conversation from "What's wrong?" to "What is needed to bring well-being to my web of meaning?" However, what is wrong, and what we say about it, can often give us clues about what we need.

There are lots of systems that present maps of meaning based on where illness shows up in the body. For example, in Chinese medicine, meridians serve as energy streams that each support and feed not only an organ but the energy represented by it. The heart meridian supports the heart as an organ and also your ability to connect with others. The stomach meridian supports not only the stomach as an organ but your ability to embody and cope with experiences in the world. If you know some of these body and energy mapping systems, you can more easily recognize what your symptoms are telling you about energy disruptions.

Even without formal maps, however, you can use language to recognize energy issues. Describe your health challenge to a friend, and record yourself talking. Then listen together with your friend to get help to hear the subtext. Here are some examples:

- If you find yourself saying, "I feel like crap," recognize what you are saying. Crap is the material we release after pulling all the nutrients from food. So the crap you are feeling is the dross: energy that is backed up or leftover. Find some gesture or energy unity that helps you to release it. Use the "Mother Teresa Touch" (page 15).
- If you say, "I'm soooo tired. I'm tired all the time," you are saying: "My actions aren't being fueled." Dialogue with your gatekeeper and assess what radiance you are pulling in to fuel your life. Use "Bringing In Your Spirit Feeds" (page 156) and "Adjusting the Flames" (page 115).
- If you say, "I'm feeling defeated," think about what alternative "feats" can be brought in to replace the ones that didn't come through.
- If your joints ache, look at ways you work with bending,

flexibility, and connection (the job of joints), and look at transitions in your day — the metaphoric joints of your schedule. Pain is almost always a signal that energy is blocked (or disconnected), so clearing that blockage with stretching, gentle movement, and other energy tools can help. Try singing your core note to remind your body of its baseline "key." Then send sound vibrating into each joint to help release or retune the energies stuck there. Try bringing some activity to clear the palate into every transition of your day: Do some artwork; take a five-minute walk; lie down; or do a few energy medicine exercises that reset your energies for the next task.

Use the symptom, its location, and behaviors as pointers to what might be healthy inputs. This makes your body feel heard, helps your mind engage in something more productive, and communicates to your soul that you are participating. Over time, you will develop your own personalized maps that help you navigate how your body uses symptoms to express your energetic needs.

CONVERSATION ONE:
GATEKEEPING — IDENTITY AND BOUNDARIES

As a reminder, the gatekeeper governs your physical, emotional, energetic, and spiritual immune system.

There is a rich literature evolving on how you can use nutrition to heal and support your immune system. There are ongoing new discoveries about the influence of your microbiome not just on gut health but also on your overall ability to thrive. As a self-healer, I have found it useful to delve into that literature and get educated. Your microbiome is the community of microorganisms found in your gut and elsewhere in your body. They can have a profound influence on your health. Estimates are that there are ten times as many microorganisms as cells living within you.[14] This biological approach is helpful, but it does not address the energetics of the immune system.

What I call the gatekeeper includes the energetic mechanisms that govern how well your immune system and your subtle energies function to create and maintain a body. In the Earth Elemental realm, the gatekeeper energetically supports your hormones to launch, your body's chemistry to hum, and your body to maintain its integrity. It also influences your microbiome.

In "A Brief Introduction to the Gatekeeper" (page 136), I point out the four main jobs of the gatekeeper:

1. **To maintain the sanctity of the self.** The priority is to keep you safe and intact, but not necessarily happy. What is in your best interest in maintaining the sanctity of that self might conflict with goals you set that you think will make you happy.

2. **To create identity.** Since the task is to help you build an understanding of what is me and not me, this becomes the basis for repelling substances and energies that threaten your identity. It is also the basis for funding or attracting energies that support your identity.

3. **To regulate the distribution of energies.** Your gatekeeper determines what gets funded and what doesn't. The priorities it sets for this are safety first, then preserving and protecting identity, and then continuation of forms or habits. It doesn't like change! Only when guided by your Wiser Self via radiance will your gatekeeper fund new patterns.

4. **To keep the habits.** The gatekeeper runs your body's autopilot and autonomic nervous system, keeping the habits or templates of experience and maintaining continuity. Although the gatekeeper doesn't like change, it is a necessary participant in making change.

Since we span a spectrum of several dimensions, gatekeeping also operates not only within the body but also in the realms of the Talking Self and Wiser Self.

In the realm of Talking Self, the gatekeeper builds up a library of templates of experiences, what my inner teachers used to call *gatekeeper robots*. They operate a bit like apps on your phone. They are programmed to run the instrument and interact with the world in a certain way.

At this Talking Self level, the gatekeeper builds a composite sense of self and identity. It forms beliefs, rooted in your experiences, that influence thought, emotions, and behaviors. These, in turn, affect how your body operates. For example, if you believe that "people tend to like me," this keeps your body and mind relaxed when encountering new people. Your gatekeeper sends out energetic messages of comfort that influence people to like you.

On the other hand, if your gatekeeper has set up a template that codifies "people don't tend to like me," perhaps based on painful past experience, that sets off cascades of stress hormones in your body and communicates energetic warning to the people you meet.

When your gatekeeper is healthy, it works in close consultation with your conscious mind. It allows you to function in the present. You get ongoing insight into how your subtle energies are moving so you can co-create your experiences of mind and body.

But when your autopilot gets clogged with old templates for habits that no longer serve you, it is more likely to run the ship aground. It knocks your subtle energies off-balance, replicating your past problems or pulling you into distorted thinking about the future. And that sets the stage for physical illness and breakdown. (Use "Clearing Templates in the Chakras," page 143, for help clearing gatekeeper templates.)

At the level of the Wiser Self, the gatekeeper acts as a nudge to remind you of your soul's purpose:

- The gatekeeper communicates with your Talking Self through ideas, thoughts, emotions, images, events, urges, and feelings of aversion.
- The gatekeeper communicates with your Earth Elemental Self through symptoms, influencing the body's energy flows and creating events (such as accidents or serendipity, calling your attention to something, and behaviors that attract or repel others).

These all serve to remind the Earth Elemental Self and Talking Self of Wiser Self's perspective.

When you break out in hives, or fall down and smash your nose, it is not always clear how that supports Wiser Self's purpose. But in fact, almost all imbalance contains pointers to what balance might look like. Symptoms can awaken you to what needs to be brought more consciously into the conversation.

It is a good investment to befriend and learn to partner with your gatekeeper!

If you feel your immune system is running away with you (you experience too much emotional and physical reactivity), your gatekeeper needs some template clearing. In addition, the exercises presented to support this conversation — "Porcupine Reset" (page 201), "Yin Hearts" (page 198), and "Reinforcing the Smart Filter of the Aura" (page 205) — help you to enter into better and ongoing dialogue with your gatekeeper, giving it more up-to-date instructions on safety, identity, energy distribution, and creation of templates that reflect your inner truth.

GATEKEEPER REACTIVITY

You probably recognize gatekeeper reactivity best when symptoms get triggered, such as when you eat something and develop a rash or stomachache. But reactivity takes many forms. Somebody says something that makes your heart race as your mind forms angry retorts. You see a difficult family member and find yourself unable to concentrate afterward. Depending on what your body does to signal distress, it might be your trick knee going out, your chronic headache starting up, or even an uncomfortable social behavior, such as suddenly sounding annoyingly just like your hypercritical father.

Your gatekeeper reacts to threats or needs by destabilizing the energy flows that run your body. You are probably familiar with the concept of fight-or-flight. These are reactions of the *yang gatekeeper*, which maintains your relationships with the world. When the yang gatekeeper is triggered, it usually releases a cascade of stress hormones to prepare you to fight or get yourself out of the situation.

The *yin gatekeeper* has another task: to protect the experience of your soul being embodied, the sanctity of your self. The yin gatekeeper signals when something violates your inner truth or threatens your heart in some way. Yin gatekeeper reactivity takes the forms of *freeze or fog*.

Freeze is what a deer does in the headlights. In humans, it can also take the form of physical, emotional, or mental shutdown. Fog is what squid or skunks do. They put out something to muddle the senses. In humans, fogging can involve becoming vague or scrambled. It can also involve inarticulate speech or compulsive talking that obscures the conversation. Yin fogging can happen energetically, apparently invisibly, when everyone in the room is suddenly confused or scrambled because someone in that room has gone into yin gatekeeper reactivity and fogged the space.

• • • EXERCISE: YIN HEARTS • • •

For yin gatekeeper reactivity, try this exercise:

Slowly and lovingly trace at least three hearts over your physical heart, or over any body part that needs it. It is especially helpful to do this motion touching the skin with moderate pressure, so you connect with the skin layer called the *fascia*, if possible. This communicates the loving, calming energy via the crystalline structure built into your fascia, which serves as a body-wide rapid communication pathway.

"Yin Hearts" is so simple, it may appear to be just a little self-love gesture. But our subtle energies work via the principle of resonance as well as influence; they can impact one another even when they aren't physically connected. So this exercise can:

- clear blockages of yin energy coming in from both earth and sky
- help the heart and intuition to open
- even help calm the vagus nerve, a physiological pathway used by the yin gatekeeper to register any reactivity that is geared to protect the sanctity of the self

As you tune in to the yin gatekeeper energies via this exercise, invite your heart to show you what it is yearning for, perhaps with images or words. Offer in turn your own energetic gifts to your heart, streaming them from the centers of your palms and your fingertips into the gesture.

• • • • • •

Your gatekeeper works extensively via the body's electromagnetics — its polarities. The electrical communications of the body use plus-minus signaling, like the positive-and-negative poles of a battery. Most of the energy systems of the body have positive and negative polarities as well. Your body is designed to align energetically with the north and south polarities of the earth.

When you place the north side of one magnet next to the south side of another, they attract. When you place the north side of one magnet near the north side of another, the energies repel. Your gatekeeper uses this phenomenon to flip energies when it goes into reactivity. It causes some to repel, and others to stick or glom, where they should be flowing. *The gatekeeper uses electromagnetic polarities and partitions to keep you safe!*

The gatekeeper frequently flips polarities in the aura, your energy container. It can set up energetic baffles to repel unwanted influences by creating areas of reverse polarities.

Porcupine Reactivity

Porcupine reactivity is a form of yang gatekeeper reactivity where the levels of the aura closest to the body flip their electromagnetic direction. This sends energies outward to protect your shields from perceived threats, and it can influence polarities in other levels of the aura as well. Unfortunately, since so much energy is going outward for protection, this is like in *Star Trek* when the captain sends energy to protect the shields from Klingons, causing the replicators and ship maintenance systems to falter. Flipped polarities cause your life support systems (digestion, circulation, tissue repair, and so on) to go on brownout and malfunction. In the aura, it looks something like the image in figure 18.

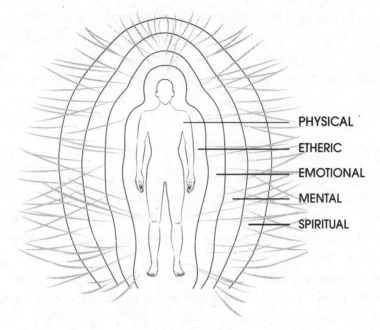

PHYSICAL

ETHERIC

EMOTIONAL

MENTAL

SPIRITUAL

Figure 18. Porcupine reactivity in the aura

I first noticed this in someone who was prickly, quick to anger, reactive to what other people said, contentious, and just plain uncomfortable to be around. As I looked at her, I realized that she had a flipped polarity in one of the layers of her aura that made her look energetically like a porcupine with quills fully extended! It occurred to me that if she could be helped to retract her quills, people would feel more comfortable around her and she would feel less endangered.

I taught her an exercise I created, "Porcupine Reset" (below), and it was something of a miracle cure. It caused an immediate shift in her inner and outer presence. When her polarity reversed, the energy quills retracted, and her whole energy communication transformed. She was pleasant, relaxed, and had a lovely sense of humor. This was a great relief for both of us.

It took her some time, using "Porcupine Reset" frequently, until she could train her gatekeeper to change the habit of such strong reactivity in her aura. But at least she had a tool to make that change, and eventually, she became a consistently more comfortable person, within herself and in her interactions with others.

• • • EXERCISE: PORCUPINE RESET • • •

To support your yang gatekeeper and pull it out of porcupine reactivity, the correction is simple, like turning an inside-out sock right side out. You first bring "sky energy" down from the top of your head in an egg-shaped arc. Tack that energy to the ground, then pull "earth energy" up from beside your feet in an egg-shaped arc and tack it to the top of your head. The full movement looks like figure 19.

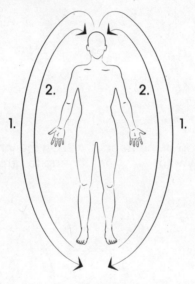

Figure 19. Porcupine Reset overview

Here is a step-by-step guide:

1. Starting at the top of the head, grab the energy with two hands.
2. On the inhale, pull it straight up to arm's length.
3. On the exhale, pull it down on either side of your body, arcing out (egg-shaped arc).
4. Tack the energy to the floor.
5. Grab energy from the earth.
6. On the inhale, pull it up with both hands, arcing out.
7. On the exhale, tack it to the top of the head.

See figure 20 for a detailed step-by-step illustration of the movements.

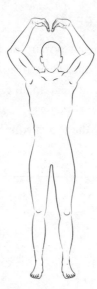
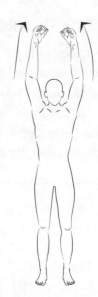

1. Starting at the top of the head, grab the energy with two hands.

2. On the inhale, pull it straight up to arm's length.

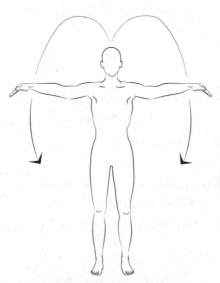
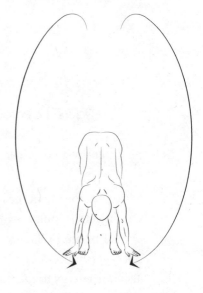

3. On the exhale, pull it down on either side of your body, arcing out (egg-shaped arc).

4. Tack the energy to the floor.

Figure 20. Porcupine Reset step-by-step movements

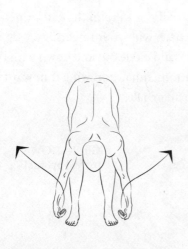

5. Grab energy from the earth.

6. On the inhale, pull it up with both hands, arcing out.

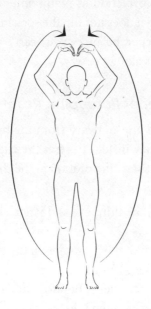

7. On the exhale, tack it to the top of the head.

Porcupine Reset on an Organ

To pull an organ out of gatekeeper reactivity or to calm the gatekeeper in a particular location, trace the same pattern with your fingers:

Start at the top of that organ, inhale, and circle out and down with the exhale. Then grab the energy at the bottom, inhale, drawing it upward in a semicircle, and tack it to the top with an exhale.

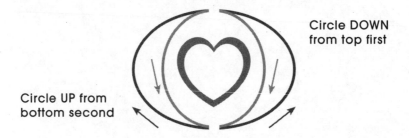

Circle DOWN from top first

Circle UP from bottom second

Figure 21. Porcupine Reset on an organ

You can repeat this correction as many times as necessary. After the first correction, repeating it does not flip the sock inside out again! Instead it calms the yang gatekeeper, balances your earth and sky, and generally corrects flipped polarities along the way.

Inner Porcupine Reset

The aura extends inward and outward from the body, so this correction helps when you feel prickly inside. To reset the energy, do the same kind of egg-shaped action, but start the motion at the third eye:

1. Pull energy from the third eye and stretch arms upward with the inhale.
2. Arc out and down to the ground with the exhale and tack the "sky energy" to the ground.
3. Then grasp the earth energy beside your feet and pull upward in an outward arc with the inhale.
4. Tack it to your third eye with the exhale.

• • • • • •

These exercises are very simple to do. However, remember, you can use them to tune in and *assess* what is happening with your gatekeeper, *rebalance* the energies through the motion, and if your gatekeeper could use more resources, *invoke* a quality (such as deep peace or safety) and infuse that quality from your hands into your gatekeeper as you do the exercise.

• • • EXERCISE: REINFORCING • • •
THE SMART FILTER OF THE AURA

Try this exercise for building safety and clearer boundaries:

At the edge of the aura (your energy field) is a filter that determines what can come in and what goes out. It serves as a boundary or container for your subtle energies. I call it the "smart filter" because it is a programmable feature of your gatekeeper (and thus, it is *smart*). When you strengthen and reinforce your smart filter, you reinforce the boundary between *me* and *not me* and teach your gatekeeper more balanced ways to interact with the world. Your gatekeeper learns from this, and even pulls energies out of your field that no longer fit with the *me* you are reinforcing.

With your arms extended, use your radiant imagination to send figure eights out to the edge of your aura. Because the aura fluctuates in size, between being close to the body to extending beyond the limits of the room, you need to use your imagination and intention to aim for the present edge of your aura. The figure-eight motion you use is toward your body and away from it, since you are figure-eighting between what is you and what is not you at the edge of your field.

Figure-eighting the edge of the aura helps to create balance between the energies of your own aura and the energies of other fields, so that the passage between those two is smooth and balanced.

You can also do this exercise for another person, with their permission.

Since the aura is so large, like a big egg surrounding you, it's great to call on help to figure-eight the entire surface. Most clients giggle when I suggest bringing in fairies or elves or UPS delivery guys to help reinforce the edge of the aura. But doing this activates radiant energy on behalf of the process and makes it work even better. The helpers can finish up or come in periodically to help you reinforce the smart filter when you aren't able to figure-eight your own aura.

Then, fill the smart filter with a color (of your choice) using radiant imagination — and your hands — to distribute the color. Pure white light is *not* recommended for the smart filter, since it will attract lost souls (they head for the white light). If you want white, put a tint in it!

Reinforcing the smart filter can work even when someone else is standing in your energy field. Your aura is designed to intermingle with other energy fields but still hold its integrity and identity. So this exercise will key your gatekeeper to be more skilled in recognizing the *me* and the *not me*. When the smart filter is strong and is operating properly, not only will it repel or not get attached to passing energies that don't belong in your container of self, it will also gather up and spit out unwanted influences that have infiltrated your energy field.

As you assess your smart filter, tune in to whether it is robust and strong or full of holes and leaky. The more you reinforce your smart filter, the stronger your energetic boundaries and filtering become. Remember, in addition to infusing the smart filter with color, you can infuse it with energetic truths that are core to your identity.

• • • • • •

Other Exercises That Support the Gatekeeper

Most of the exercises in this book help calm your gatekeeper because the gatekeeper's job is to signal energy needs. However, these exercises are especially helpful:

Clear Fear, Ease Ego, Welcome Wiser Self (page 148)
Divine Hook-Up (page 139)
Adjusting the Flames (page 115)
Seven Spirals (page 225)
Core Note (page 96)
Sing a Scale (page 222)
Cabinets of Wonders (page 79)
Core Shape (page 109)
Bringing In Your Spirit Feeds (page 156)
Dumbo (page 234)
Mother Teresa Touch (page 15)
Full-Body Grounding and Rooting (page 209)
The Four Stabilizing Colors (page 86)

CONVERSATION TWO:
GROUNDING, ROOTING, AND ANCHORING

Grounding goes beyond whether your feet are planted solidly on the earth. You are energetically grounded, rooted, and anchored in a number of ways: via your connection to the planet; via your spiritual roots; via your air roots out into the environment; via your connections with people, ideas, communities, rituals, and habits; and via your elemental nature.

We often use the term *grounding* to refer to three different energetic tasks:

Grounding is my ability to return unwanted energies to the earth, as in a grounding wire.

Rooting is my ability to connect to something and get nourishment, the way a tree sends roots into the soil or a plant in water sends out hydroponic roots.

Anchoring is my ability to attach to something that keeps me oriented and steady, the way a boat is anchored to keep it in the harbor.

Although we sometimes use these words interchangeably when we speak, in energetic terms they represent three interrelated issues.

Lack of grounding, rooting, and anchoring — or faulty connections in these three processes — often underlies chronic energy imbalance and the stress that creates dysfunction. It is usually part of any acute or chronic illness. Therefore, cultivating healthy grounding, roots, and anchors is part of an ongoing conversation of well-being.

Grounding

If grounding is the connection that allows your energies to return to the earth, or to be wicked off so they don't back up in the system, it is clear why grounding is important.

You need to be able to use energy and then let it go, like your body processes food and eliminates the parts that don't serve you. When energies back up in the system, you are likely to feel it in your nerves, and it affects your body-mind communications. Children who have ADD and can't concentrate often have an issue with grounding their energies back to Source. They need regular movement to help them wick off the excess energy so it doesn't overwhelm the body's circuits. They need contact not only with the earth but with activities or environments that can help to draw off the excess charge.

Consider what it does to children with inadequate grounding to sit still in a classroom, trying to organize the energetic inputs around them. The energies building up in their system have no outlet. That causes the mind to skip, the gatekeeper to trigger reactivity, and the nervous system to misfire. Calming the nervous system with medications begs the question of how to teach children to wick off unneeded energies.

Ironically, for some children with ADD, playing video games (a stimulating activity) helps them to concentrate. The stimulation helps them build up steam, which then has enough pressure to trigger release. The games also provide outlets for their pent-up nervous energy to clear out, grounding them. Whether this is the healthiest form of grounding is a question, but it does the trick.

As you assess your grounding, you can tune in to whether energies enter your system and exit again with good rhythms and ease. This includes looking at whether you take food in, metabolize it, and eliminate it in comfortable patterns. Whether you draw breath in and release it fully. And whether you draw in vital force to fuel a task, use it to complete that task, and then are able to let the activity go afterward. Can you listen to a friend, take in what they are saying, respond, then let go of the conversation? Can you participate in an event, let it stimulate and enrich you, then ground the energies back to the earth or into some other realm at the end?

In other words, grounding, while being focused on the *release* of energies, helps you to participate in cycles of both activity and rest. Without adequate grounding, these cycles are disrupted and disrupt the health of your body, emotions, and relationships. They skew your choices.

We are grounded by having outlets. Here are some basic ones:

First, you need a good connection with the earth, so you can give back energies, thoughts, and vibrations you don't need to keep active in your system.

Second, you need ways to release excess stimulation from energies backed up in your body, to shake them off the way a rabbit that escapes being run over can go under a bush and just shake until the adrenaline effect calms. Shaking your stress off is a good tool to use for yourself. Shaking that comes from within can help the gatekeeper let go of reactivity. However, please be aware that shaking others, particularly infants, can do harm.

Third, you need movement, not just in the form of a monster workout in the morning, but throughout the day. Muscles bunch and take on energetic signals, and they need to release that energy in an ongoing way through gentle movements, swaying, walking, moving the arms in figure-eight patterns, fidgeting, and so on.

Fourth, you need healthy exhales. The exhale grounds you.

Fifth, you need places to put your energies. You are grounded by engagement in situations that allow you to contribute, not just participate. Energies that enter your web of meaning are grounded by being shared with others in meaningful ways!

• • • EXERCISE: FULL-BODY GROUNDING • • • AND ROOTING

This exercise is great to do if you are feeling overwhelmed, overloaded, or pent up, or if you are confused about what energy medicine is needed. Like "Mother Teresa Touch" (page 15), it can give you a whole-system reset.

Lie facedown on the earth or the floor and just allow all the confusion and energy and thought to drain back into the earth. Give it all over to mother earth. (If this is too difficult for you physically, you can do it on a bed.) A whole-body plant on the earth allows you to ground with every cell of your body.

Turn over onto your back and send all the excess energies from your back and spine down into the earth.

Send roots down from every vertebra of your spine and from every cell on the back of your body, paying special attention to the sacrum. Lie there until you feel the roots bringing nourishment up into your system. Open the front of your body and allow sky energy to stream down into you and through you, mixing and balancing with the earth energies coming in via your roots.

• • • • • •

Rooting

Once you recognize that rooting is the act of pulling in nourishment, it is easy to see that you need to root into more than just mother earth. You need to root into the *sky* energies, into your own core self, into the elemental rhythms, and into a storyline that fits your nature and instrument.

Like a plant, we put out connectors that pull nutrients from the soil where we are planted. I believe we are energetically fed (or malnourished) by the geography of the land where we live. For many people, the landscape where they grew up nourishes them. For others, it sends their gatekeeper into reactivity. You have to determine for yourself: Does the land you are living on feed you? How does the geography influence your subtle energies? I've lived in a lot of places over time, and some of the places drained me and left me feeling like a beached whale; others overstimulated my body's electrics; and others felt like home, the right feel to nourish my body and keep my rhythms humming.

Your memberships in your family, through your work and friendships, in your community and society, similarly act as roots bringing in energetic nourishment (or poisons).

The elements of nature nourish us via the foods we eat. We are nourished by the sun, wind, water, and electromagnetic rhythms via our encounters with nature.

If you are aware of your roots, you begin to think of wellness in terms of what nourishes you and what poisons your own personal well.

Energy medicine can support the establishment of healthy rooting, but in addition, I turn to *lifestyle medicine* activities that feed and nourish me, that root me in this existence. Reading a book nourishes me. Washing dishes grounds me and roots me because having my hands in water and scrubbing releases excess energy. The water itself, and the satisfaction of getting pots clean, nourishes me. Grocery shopping energizes me, but it drains my partner's energies. Therefore, establishing and tending to your root system, your connection to the world around you, is a very individualized wellness practice. Of course, grounding, rooting, and anchoring sometimes happen within a single activity.

Anchoring

Anchors are habits or attachments that feed our sense of orientation in life. Healthy anchors differ from individual to individual. For one person, an anchor may be a morning ritual; for another, it may be a favorite piece of clothing or a comfort food. For others, it may be a song, a job, a role, an identity, or a certain activity.

My house and neighborhood anchor me. My birth identity anchors me in a group or history that sometimes conflicts with some of my chosen affiliations. My friendship with one person keeps me part of a social group but may prevent my membership in another. My body anchors my attention in the here or now, while my Talking Self identities allow me to travel to specific imaginary spaces that anchor me in conceptual frameworks and more abstract realms. All membership is an anchor. Some memberships also act as roots bringing in nourishment or providing a release that grounds us.

An anchor is not just an emotional bond. It is energetic. It can affect your subtle energies, supporting well-being or illness.

Your web of meaning is part of a larger exchange of energies. Anchors are the energetic bonds you set up to keep you entrained or attached to situations or people. They keep you feeling secure and oriented. If anchors are missing or unhealthy, the gatekeeper gets triggered and will signal its discomfort via symptoms and reactivity. For example, if your attachment to a partner limits your life so much that you can't live your soul's truth, this will trigger your gatekeeper to express its needs via symptoms.

Anchoring in other people or creatures can be either helpful or disruptive, depending on the nature of the bond and relationship. And when you lose a beloved anchor (a pet, a person, a job), it is crucial that you find yourself new moorings to support your wellness.

The model for a healthy anchor is the bonding that happens between mother and infant when that relationship is positive and interactive. If you didn't get that healthy bonding as a child, your key to self-healing is likely to include cultivating healthy anchors, rooting, and grounding. Most important in self-healing is to establish an anchor in your own physical being. That usually includes some sensorimotor reworking of your instrument (see "Sensorimotor," page 39).

As you grow up, your gatekeeper continuously identifies people, places, sounds, smells, sensations, beliefs, and substances it deems safe and nourishing, based on both active experience and inborn predilections. These become your personalized anchors for nourishment of your body's energies. (If these are not healthy anchors, you will need to do some template clearing; see "Clearing Templates in the Chakras," page 143).

Healthy anchors are personal to you: whatever nourishes you and helps you stay grounded. Unhealthy anchors are any attachment that interferes with your ability to ground or root.

• • • EXERCISE: EARTH DOCK–SKY DOCK • • •

This exercise helps to ground, root, and anchor you between earth, sky, and the five elements of your nature, raising your vibration.

Earth Docking

Many of us are feeling unstable, ill at ease, ungrounded, and emotionally or socially shaky these days. We are experiencing upheaval in aspects of our inner or outer life we believed to be secure.

Although these feelings affect us personally, it may not be personal. The earth's electromagnetic field is fluctuating more rapidly and erratically as of late. It can feel as if we are on the deck of a ship, pitching and rolling in a storm.

This is a simple technique for getting your taproots planted into a secure source. Taproots are an energetic feature that extends downward from the foot at the kidney 1 (K-1) point (see figures 22 and 23). They can be seen as part of the root chakra, extending downward beyond the body.

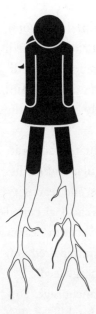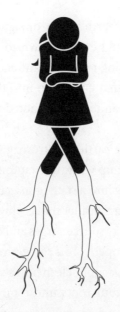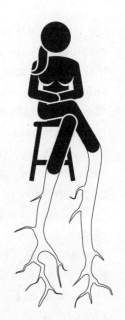

Figure 22. Taproots

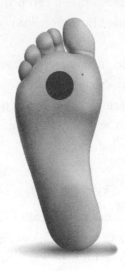

Figure 23. The K-1 point

Historically (until the earth's electromagnetics became less stable), each person's taproots would extend down to the level below the earth that had the most nourishing and resonant energy source for each individual. They would bring that energy up into the body via the K-1 point through the kidney meridian to be distributed to the body by way of the meridian system.

Now, however, with the earth's electromagnetics fluctuating so erratically, the energy you bring up with your taproots is irregular and/or disturbed. It throws your body into a state of insecurity, stress, and reactivity.

It is like having a vacuum cleaner that is plugged into a short-circuited electrical outlet; as the energy source surges and drops, the vacuum cleaner stutters and won't work properly. You can get your vacuum repaired, but the problem isn't with the vacuum cleaner; it's with the energy feed!

So it is crucial to get your roots into a more stable anchorage. Fortunately, we have such an anchorage. It is an energetically stabilized *shelf* that sits about eight feet below the surface of the earth.

The shelf is like a computer docking station. It is connected up to all the earth's energetic strata, so that it can bring us the earth nourishment we need, but in a stabilized form. You just need to plug your taproots into it.

Inhale, and on the exhale, imagine sending your taproots down from the kidney 1 point (a one-inch circle on the bottom of each foot; see figure 23) till they reach eight feet below the surface of the earth to connect with the shelf, aka the earth dock. You can usually sense when the taproots click into connection with the earth dock.

Sky Docking

Once you have earth docked, use your breath to help pull the energy up through your body (inhale), out the top of your head (exhale), and anchor it in the star that has your name on it — your soul's star.

As with earth docking, sky docking can be visualized as a *sky root* or just seen as an energetic handshake.[15]

Feel that connection for a few seconds. Use your breath to feel the sky-docked energy travel down to and through the top of your head (inhale), through your body (exhale), and out your feet, so that it anchors back at the earth dock.

Earth docking and sky docking can be done in any position, but if you are standing with your legs somewhat apart, you can feel the energies anchoring you into what I call your "power triangle."

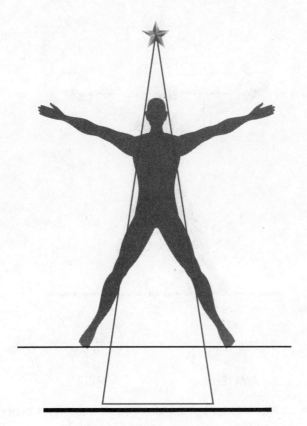

Figure 24. The Power Triangle

This is your most grounded power base from which to do energy medicine.

When your sky dock is linked with the earth dock, bring that connected energy to your heart by placing both palms on your heart.

Balancing Your Earth-Docked, Sky-Docked Energies

If you stretch your arms out to each side, you will see that you are in fact a five-element star (for more on this, see "Elemental Balance," page 174).

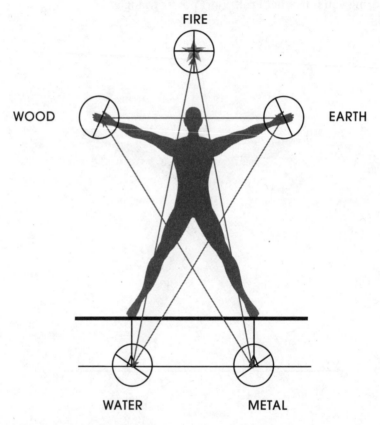

Figure 25. Earth-docked, sky-docked five-element balance

In this position, the five elements are as follows:

- **Water:** below the right foot at the earth dock
- **Metal:** below the left foot at the earth dock
- **Wood:** right hand
- **Earth:** left hand
- **Fire:** above the head at the sky dock

In this position, you can reinforce the control and flow cycles of your earth-docked and sky-docked self. First, use figure eights to trace the control cycle along the five-pointed star (figure-eighting between water and fire, between fire and metal, between metal and wood, between wood and earth, and between earth and water). Then figure-eight the flow cycle in a clockwise circle around the points (from water to wood, wood to fire, fire to earth, earth to metal, metal to water).

Or, as an alternative, to reinforce the flow, just circle your arm three to four times in the direction of the flow cycle. Then end by placing your hand on your heart to ground your heart as well.

This exercise can be done quickly to ground, root, and anchor you in multiple dimensions. Or it can be done more slowly and used to tune in to your earth/sky balance (feet and head), to assess your *outreach* energies (left and right hands), and to feel the interrelationship between your elements as you trace the five-pointed star. Invoke whatever qualities you wish, including such phrases as: "May I know grace," "May I dwell in peace," "May I be filled with kindness," or "May I know my powers."

• • • • • •

Other Exercises That Support Grounding, Rooting, and Anchoring

In addition to these exercises, drinking water can also ground and root you.

Seven Spirals (page 225)
The Four Stabilizing Colors (page 86)
Five-Element Bed or Chair (page 176)
Bringing In Your Spirit Feeds (page 156)
Core Note (page 96)
Divine Hook-Up (page 139)
Go with the Flow — The K-27 Thump (page 101)
Yin Hearts (page 198)
Aligning the Three Selves (page 135)
Cosmic Figure Eight (page 158)

PRACTICE TIPS

- When you are feeling ill, explore how you can love up your body, mind, and spirit the way you would an ailing family pet.
- Look at ways that perfectionism turns your self-care into self-tyranny. Are you listening and responding to your body's communications moment by moment or following rules someone (including you) has set for you? Practice energy dialogue regularly for a period of a week or two in place of trying to implement a scripted wellness program.
- As you revisit the exercises in this book, do them in such a way that you first tune in, then assess, then invoke desired qualities, rather than just doing them as you might do jumping jacks.
- Explore what your illness and symptoms can teach you, or what your body might be communicating via the discomfort. Listen to the language you use to describe how you feel, as that often gives you clues to what is happening or what is needed.
- Make friends with your gatekeeper. How is it operating in your life? If you are experiencing lots of reactivity, calm the gatekeeper reactions using the exercises presented in this book. Then look more deeply at what kind of support your yang and yin gatekeepers need to keep you safe and whole.
- Explore how grounding, rooting, and anchoring play out specifically for you and contribute to chronic illness or imbalance.

Chapter Eleven

CULTIVATING WELLNESS

When you get sick, it is tempting to look outside yourself for causes: germs, microorganisms, toxins in the environment, events that cause you stress, or your relationships. While these all can be instrumental in catalyzing illness, more often there are underlying issues within your construction of self that trigger your gatekeeper to cascade into immune system reactivity and symptoms. These include how well you:

- are gatekeeping your energy dance
- are grounded, rooted, and anchored
- are holding together within yourself and experiencing coherence
- are holding your own in response to encounters with the world
- are having a healthy energy flow and exchange within you
- are accessing radiance, the energy that animates you and brings you into true well-being

The first two on this list are addressed in conversations one and two (chapter 10). In this chapter, the rest of these issues are explored with a focus on how they support wellness.

CONVERSATION THREE:
INNER CONNECTIONS AND COHERENCE

Subtle energies don't work in isolation in the body. They are part of a large, swirling, pulsing, spiraling, flowing energy exchange. They need to cooperate with one another in order to work properly.

This is easy enough to see in terms of organs. My two lungs have to entrain and work in tandem. My heart and lungs have to coordinate. My various digestive organs need to work together and communicate back and forth to get the job done.

All this coordination leads to balance within myself and a sense of coherence, my parts all working together in a unified whole.

At the root of maintaining inner coordination is staying connected within yourself. That has always been a struggle for me. I joke that I have a sticky brain because anything I see or hear just comes in and gets stuck in me. Because I get so clogged, my subtle energies react and disconnect from one another. My individual parts are working, but nothing is getting done because they aren't working together.

My stomach sends a message to my gut, but the gut doesn't hear the message, and so my stomach has to yell louder and goes into overdrive. If my body produces insulin, and the receptors on the cells are clogged and resistant, my body just pumps out more and more insulin, flooding the system. And even though allopathic medicine does recognize some of the intrabody communications that have to happen, it is not good at promoting better dialogue across organs and systems. Energy medicine, yoga, and acupuncture all support a system-wide form of inner connection and flow that needs to happen to get every part of you on the same page.

It is an important wellness dialogue to find ways to create inner connection and coherence: the rhythm that supports balance between your organs; the integrating thread that pulls your different energy systems and parts of your self into relationship; the weaving together of energies that make up your web of meaning.

If your focus is on illness, breakdown, what is wrong, pain, darkness, and defeat, chances are you aren't finding the hope, or other connective threads, needed to inspire your energies to work as a team.

What helps supply the connective thread?

- **Hook-up holds:** The most basic inner connection to look for on the physical level is to make sure that energy is hooked up: between front and back, between the left side and right side of the body, between your back brain and front brain, between your head and heart and gut, and between upper and lower body. You can use your two hands to hook up any organs or parts that need to communicate.

  If you only have the use of one hand, touch each place consecutively, then figure-eight between them. In a pinch you can use a large surface, such as a wall, bed, person, plus intention, to bridge places that need better communication. That is one reason a hug can do such a good job of supporting inner connection.

- **Figure eights:** In Eden Energy Medicine, we teach our clients to figure-eight between all parts of their body and energy field. The figure-eight shape is perhaps the most basic pattern of subtle energy movement, and Donna Eden frequently says that the more cross-over patterns she sees in a person's energy field, the healthier they are.

- **Unifying focus:** In an orchestra, the conductor unifies and coordinates all the players. In the body, the breath serves the same purpose. You can also use your core note, a mantra, a rhythmic pulse, or touch to bring your parts into sync.

- **Storyline:** The story you tell yourself about what is happening to you matters. Whenever we can create a narrative thread that pulls us forward, frames our situation in a positive light, or gives us a larger purpose, it tends to get the energy systems working together better. Consider the difference you are communicating to your body and gatekeeper between saying, "I'm falling apart," or "I'm losing it," and saying, "I'm disconnecting so I can reformulate."

The following two exercises will also help you with inner connection and coherence.

• • • EXERCISE: SING A SCALE • • •

Sing a scale up and down, at least two or three times. If this is challenging for you, don't worry, there are apps and YouTube videos for singing along.

Singing a scale is a *great* way to reinforce inner connection. Each note on the scale correlates with a different energy system within you. By singing the scale up and down two or three times, you are placing the systems into vibrational connection and strengthening their coherence. Try this when you are feeling scattered, conflicted, or fractionated.

• • • • • •

• • • EXERCISE: TWELVE HEARTS • • •

If you are not comfortable with sound tools, or you just want to vary your routine, try this exercise. It is adapted, with gratitude, from an Eden Energy Medicine exercise called Nine Hearts.

Start with both hands on the center of your chest, over your heart chakra. Tune in to your heart and focus for a moment on someone or something you love. Then, slowly and lovingly, draw both hands up through the midpoint of your face, and circle outward, tracing a heart around your face. Return your hands to your starting point at the heart chakra. Repeat that motion twice more, tracing a total of three hearts in that position.

Hold your heart chakra a moment to feel the love. Then trace a heart over your upper torso region, with the point of that heart at the belly button. After each tracing, return your hands to your heart chakra. Repeat that motion twice more, completing three hearts in that position.

Then shift your hands down to cover your belly button. Tune in to that area for a moment, then draw three hearts, beginning at the belly button and circling down to encompass your pelvic bowl, with the point of your heart at your root chakra, then return your hands to center on your belly button. Repeat that motion twice more, completing three hearts in that position.

Finally, bring your hands back to your heart chakra. Trace a giant heart around your whole body, with arms reaching out to encompass your entire aura, and the point of the heart embedded within the earth. Return your hands to the heart chakra, then trace two more full-body hearts, ending the exercise with your hands on your heart chakra.

Both of these exercises deepen when you can tune in, do them in a manner that feels right for you, and invoke whatever integrative threads or vision that help you bring your selves and all your parts into coherence.

• • • • • •

Other Exercises That Support Inner Connections and Coherence

Take the concepts of connection and coherence into your life:

Doodling connected shapes, weaving, knitting, and braiding activities all support inner connection. Crossing your arms and legs or interlacing fingers while sitting also help, as does a "belly button–third eye Hook-Up" (page 131).

Healing Hands (page 74)
Core Note (page 96)
Core Shape (page 109)
Harmonizing Hook-Up (page 235)
Aligning the Three Selves (page 135)
Go with the Flow — The K-27 Thump (page 101)
Cabinets of Wonders (page 79)
Porcupine Reset (page 201)
Adjusting the Flames (page 115)
Yin Hearts (page 198)
Cosmic Figure Eight (page 158)
Mother Teresa Touch (page 15)
Suit Reboot (page 230)
Five-Element Bed or Chair (page 176)

CONVERSATION FOUR:
EXCHANGE BETWEEN SELF AND WORLD

We are designed to be a part of a larger web of connections, a social, energetic exchange. If you fall out of that web of connections, you can easily become sick or lose your perspective. Your energies become malnourished in multiple ways.

If you are a self-healer, this is an especially important concept. Chronic illness is not just something that goes wrong in your own system and body. When you go to the doctor for tests, the doctor probably doesn't run checks on your family, workplace, and the people in your sphere and culture to see if the imbalance is larger than just your own functions. Imbalance and resulting health challenges can arise from energetic influences in your environment and in your relationships with other people. If you are lacking fulfilling, wholesome social exchanges, have a history of traumas with other people, or feel your membership is not legitimized, you may need to find fruitful or safe ways to rework your energetic exchanges with other people and sentient beings (like cats and dogs) as part of your healing conversation.

Buddhists call this concept *right relationship* with the world. How do I harmonize with the world around me, with other people, with the environments that influence me, and with the different thought forms and belief systems that affect me?

I also think of it as your nourishment in the world. Your give-and-take with your environment, and with others, can nourish or starve you, can steady you or leave you unbalanced.

Your mind, body, and spirit are energetically influenced by your context, by other creatures, and by your environment. Your energy field takes in environmental and relational energies and has to know how to engage in give-and-take (rather than swinging between inundation or drainage).

It takes some skill to learn how to participate in the rough and tumble of the world and then to reset your balance energetically in an ongoing way. The following exercise helps you do that. It is based on the notion that most spiritual traditions create a sacred space by invoking and creating balance within seven sacred directions.

• • • EXERCISE: SEVEN SPIRALS • • •

This exercise is particularly good for balancing or resetting the body's electrics and nervous system and for shifting persistent homolateral states (lack of cross-overs and weak figure-eight movements).

The "seven spirals" refer to the seven directions used in most sacred traditions: in front, behind, to the left, to the right, above, below, and within. You will be circling with the palm facing each direction in turn.

First, *in front of you*, circle your hand, palm facing forward. Circle in either a clockwise or counterclockwise direction, whichever feels more comfortable. Circle with your hand for seven to twelve rotations (until you feel done). Then circle the opposite way for seven to twelve rotations.

Then, *to the left of you*, do the same: circle first one way, then the other, starting either clockwise or counterclockwise, whichever feels most comfortable.

Proceed through each direction, circling first one way, then the opposite, each time with your palm facing in that direction: *to the right of you, behind you, above you, below you*, and then *within*. For *within*, it usually feels good to make circles on the chest around the heart.

By doing this, you are aligning yourself with each sacred direction and reestablishing your harmony with the universe. It resets your energies for a balanced give-and-take with the world.

In this exercise, tuning in and assessing the energies of each direction can give you rich information. Notice which directions are challenging or easy, clogged or flowing. In rough terms, in front of you is where you are headed, and behind is where you have been. The left is your receptive, yin side; the right is your more active, yang side. Above is your sky feed, cosmic energies. Below is your earth feed, embodiment energies. And within is the contribution of your own inner truth and heart.

• • • • • •

> ### Other Exercises That Help Reestablish Balance with the World
>
> Cosmic Figure Eight (page 158)
> Reinforcing the Smart Filter of the Aura (page 205)
> Bringing In Your Spirit Feeds (page 156)
> Cabinets of Wonders (page 79)
> Earth Dock–Sky Dock (page 212)
> Porcupine Reset (page 201)
> Yin Hearts (page 198)
> Five-Element Bed or Chair (page 176)
> The Four Stabilizing Colors (page 86)

CONVERSATION FIVE: ENERGY FLOW RESET

We are each a moving miracle, not a fixed state. The subtle energies of your body are in constant motion. They move in somewhat consistent patterns and pathways but interact in varying rhythms and unique dynamics.

Your subtle energies need space to move. When we get tight or contracted, this impedes their flow and results in pain and lowered physical functioning. Breathing, stretching, and gentle movements all help create space to support your subtle energies to flow and circulate. Your health is constantly renewed through the movements of subtle energies; they are the threads you use to weave your web of meaning.

A Brief Guide to Subtle Energy Movements

Subtle energies are designed to move in certain patterns that are good to recognize if you want to dialogue with them and use your hands and energy medicine to support them.

Up and Down

Subtle energies move in a general pattern up the front of your body and outward from your shoulder to your fingertips on the insides of your arms. Then they move from fingertips to shoulders on the backs of your arms and from the top of your head down your back.

Try tracing up the front of your body, out along the inner arm, toward the shoulder along the outer arm, and down the back of your body to the ground using the palms of your hands to listen to and also support this natural pattern of flow.[16] Repeat several times.

Meridian Pathways

Within the general up and down pattern of flow, specific streams of nourishing, vitalizing energy form a circuit called *meridian pathways*. Meridians are like rivers that carry energies throughout your system to feed the organs, support the body's chemistry, and contribute to the weave of your energetic web. Search the internet for "Chinese medicine meridians" if you want a more detailed explanation or if you are unfamiliar with this concept, which is used in many modalities of healing.[17]

These energies often play specialized roles in your body's health. They fund specific organs and functions. For example, the spleen meridian funds the spleen and pancreas, but it also supports the energy of metabolizing on all levels.

Vital qi (energy) enters your body from the earth via points between the balls of your feet, moving up the center of your body via your kidney meridian pathway. That qi then is fed via the K-27 points (see "Go with the Flow — The K-27 Thump," page 101) through riverways of meridians to vitalize them. Nourishing energies also enter your body via other yin meridian pathways, then circulate and are carried downward and out via the yang meridian pathways.[18]

Chakras

There are whirling vortexes of energy all over your body, called *chakras*, spinning in and out to call energies into your energy field and carry them out again. Seven major chakras anchor into your deepest energy grid and sit along the midpoint of your body (see figure 9, page 143), and other smaller vortexes can be found on the palms of your hands and feet and elsewhere.

Circle counterclockwise with palms facing the body to help clear junk out of the chakras. Imagine the clock printed on your body to find counterclockwise. Circling clockwise, about six to twelve inches out from the body in your energy field, can reinforce their natural flow. Note: On men, the seventh chakra on top of the head may spin in a reverse pattern. If so, circling clockwise first, then counterclockwise, will help to clear it. This is an Eden Energy Medicine technique.

Auras or Energy Fields

Your subtle energies form a large field, your aura, that filters energies coming into that field and moves them via influence, resonance, and electromagnetic plus-minus signaling. The aura attracts and repels energies as needed and provides protection.

Move your hands slowly through the energies around your body, using your imagination to sense whether the aura is clogged or clear, clean or dirty, whole or leaky. Bring radiance and color and sound to reinstate a healthy atmosphere surrounding your body. Your aura should extend at least to arm's length. If it feels too extended, pull it in by using rolling motions with your hands, reeling it in closer to your body. If it is too tight, roll it outward.

Fountain of Energy

There is a fountain of energy that rises up through the legs and root chakra, through the center corridor of your spine, exits out the top of your head, and cascades down again in an arc all around you to bathe your energy field. It spirals out of the sacrum to ground you. When the fountain is working well, you will feel more comfortable and outgoing.

Use your hands to trace the pathway of the fountain, and as you cascade the energies around you, invoke whatever earth resources your creative self needs. Infuse this action with radiance.

Circulation of Light

There are energies that circulate in both directions up and down the spine (inside it and around it), which are sometimes called the *circulation of light*, the *microcosmic orbit*, and the *macrocosmic orbit*. This flow of subtle energy nourishes and supports the electrical and nerve communications of the body.

Massage up the front of your trunk along the midline and down the back of your spine (pressing into the spaces to either side of your spine, not pressing on the bones). You may need help from a friend to reach the back, or use a towel to clear the energies, rubbing your spine in a vertical motion with the towel. Then extend your arms to each side (parallel to the ground) and circle several times forward, then back, to animate the circulation of light at your core.

Metabolizing Subtle Energies via Digestion

Nourishment derived from food and other products of the earth is converted into energy that fuels your cellular and physiological processes via your digestion. Nourishment from sunlight is brought in via the skin.

Before you eat, tune in to all the efforts that have gone into making this food available. Recognize with gratitude the natural contributions of sun, rain, and soil, and the human contributions of all those who helped to grow, cultivate, transport, and make this food available to your body. Tune in to whatever life force vitality resides in the food and invite that into your system, feeling it release as you chew and begin the process of pulling in the nutrients and metabolizing the gifts this food brings to your being.

Figure Eights

Figure eights move energies back and forth in the field, integrating and bringing unity. Trace large and small figure eights everywhere around you, from side to side across your body, at diagonals, between front and back, top and bottom, and every which way. Weave your arms back and forth as well to integrate energies. Animate the figure eights with color and sound, sensing what kind of rhythm and movement you need.

Energy Dialogue to Support Energy Flow

We are each a big energy-converting, energy-circulating project. Your health depends on those movements working the way they are designed to work.

When you are challenged, several things happen. Your energy flows can run backward, draining you and creating fatigue and faltering functions. Your gatekeeper can flip polarities, causing energies to drain or glom, freeze or fog. Leakage occurs as blocked energies take alternative pathways and sometimes don't make it to their goal. When inner coordination fails to happen, it's like trapeze artists who swing but miss their partner and find themselves dangling in space or in free fall.

Therefore, energy dialogue that supports energy flow and bolsters it will help your overall health, and sometimes it can bring nearly miraculous cures, the same way watering a plant will revitalize it, and a good tune-up will get your car running smoothly again!

Most healing traditions offer some exercises or therapeutic treatments to reset the energy flow. In yoga, the sun salutation accomplishes this, bolstered by other poses. In Eden Energy Medicine, the "Eden Daily Energy Routine" is designed to get the subtle energy flows and patterns into connection and harmony.[19] My personal go-to energy routine to get my systems humming is offered on page 238. But because stress over the years repeatedly led my energy patterns to clog and shut down, my inner teachers also offered me the following generalized exercise to reboot my system.

• • • EXERCISE: SUIT REBOOT • • •

This is a good omnibus way to release stress and reset your body's energy systems. It is done while standing. However, before starting this exercise, make sure you are in a safe space, and do the exercises "Reinforcing the Smart Filter of the Aura" (page 205) and "Porcupine Reset" (page 201) to make sure you are not in porcupine reactivity.

When you're ready, follow these steps:

1. Imagine your body is a suit, like a big snowsuit.
2. Unzip it down the front, spread the flaps.
3. Step forward, so the suit is standing behind you. Turn to face the suit you have left standing there.

4. Lean down to pick it up by the feet. Shake it out gently like shaking wrinkles out of laundry.

5. If you wish, dip the suit in the "Well of Resolution" (or in a well filled with whatever quality you desire, such as mercy, gratitude, love).

6. Set the suit back on its feet, smoothing up the legs and arms to make sure it is upright and open for you. Then turn, step back into your suit, and zip it up!

Note: Never abandon this exercise midstream. If you need to stop, jump back in your suit quickly before moving to something else. I once had a client who was midway through it and had removed her suit, and then she heard a dogfight outside. She ran out to help, and unfortunately, she forgot to reinstate her suit. Her entire energy system was wonky and she felt dizzy and disoriented for several days until she realized what had happened and could reinstate her suit to its proper place.

• • • • • •

Other Exercises That Help Reset Energy Flow

Mother Teresa Touch (page 15)

Bringing In Your Spirit Feeds (page 156)

Core Note (page 96)

Earth Dock–Sky Dock (page 212)

Full-Body Grounding and Rooting (page 209)

Go with the Flow — The K-27 Thump (page 101)

Porcupine Reset (page 201)

Cosmic Figure Eight (page 158)

Five-Element Bed or Chair (page 176)

Harmonizing Hook-Up (page 235)

Seven Spirals (page 225)

Twelve Hearts (page 222)

Yin Hearts (page 198)

CONVERSATION SIX: BRINGING IN RADIANCE

Although the *Oxford English Dictionary* defines *radiance* as "light or heat as emitted or reflected by something," in terms of the self, radiance is much more than that. Radiance is the light of your spirit, the warmth of your vitality being expressed in your body and mind.

In young children, I have always jokingly called our capacity for radiance the "glee factor." Some babies arrive full of animation, their spirit evident in all that they do, and people respond to them readily. Other babies seem like they are not all there or are so difficult to console that the adults in their life are not as able, or motivated, to interact with them. It is all too easy for those children to fall through the cracks and fail to thrive.

All babies have some radiance, some life force "emitted or reflected" in them. They can't survive without it. But it is a capacity that you can grow and cultivate, just as you develop language, learn to relate to people, and evolve in being able to engage in this world. Though some young children are born more gleeful than others, all children deserve the loving, connected parenting that animates radiance and grows their glee factor.

Fast-forward to yourself as an adult. How well are you able to embody the radiance of your spirit, your nature? If you are struggling with chronic illness, you might find you are just treading water, getting by, rather than truly engaging with life, even on your good days. If so, cultivating your glee factor and working to access your radiance might be the missing piece.

Eileen spent years trying to heal. She studied half a dozen healing modalities, worked on herself for hours each day, consulted practitioner after practitioner. With time, her functional medicine blood tests showed balance, and her meridians and chakras were moving correctly. She had very few symptoms to complain about. And she thought this would make her happy, but it didn't. She was still just going through the motions of her life. She knew that she was no longer sick, but she also knew she wasn't well.

Eileen was suffering from a low level of radiance and an inability to assimilate and embody it. She didn't know how to enjoy her existence here on planet earth. Think about the word *enjoy*: it means to bring in joy, to give joy to. She had enough vital energy to fuel her body and allow her to move from activity to activity. But she had never developed her glee factor, her ability to use her experiences to create meaning.

Your radiance will look different from someone else's radiance. Radiance is not always loud. Think of the shimmer at dusk, quiet beauty that is a reflection of the sun's retreat. Radiance is not always outwardly focused. Think of the deep concentration on the face of a chess master. The exercises to identify your spirit feeds in chapter 8 can help you get a clearer sense of what you might do to cultivate your own style of radiance.

Like the warmth and light of the sun, radiance can seep into you in various ways. You can get *vibrational* nutrients via your spirit feeds, your energetic spine, your chakras, your meridians, your multidimensional grounding, your aura, and your exchanges with others.

I like to ask clients how well-nourished they feel. At first, they usually talk about what food they eat and how healthy it is. But that is not the point. Nourishment is a state of having *received* nutrients, metabolized them, and transformed them for use. It's not just about inputs. Nourishment comes not only from food but from all of your energetic exchanges. Think about a moment when you were exhausted and felt empty. Then you saw something funny and laughed yourself back into an energized state.

Radiance is both practical and spiritual in nature. And it is definitely a topic that deepens your ability to cultivate well-being in the face of any illness, life challenge, or malfunction.

Bringing in radiance is one of the best ways to address both illness and wellness. It enables you to dissolve and reformulate in line with deeper truths. It allows you to amplify the urgings of your Wiser Self. And it allows you to grow your glee factor. Here are three exercises designed to help you cultivate radiance.

• • • EXERCISE: JUICING WITH RADIANCE • • •

Use the "Divine Hook-Up" (page 139). Plug one index finger into a source of radiance, and then feed that radiance into any energy system or organ, like putting gas in your tank. Radiance makes everything run smoother.

Radiance, in my view, is not just a generic glow. It comes in many flavors. You can get creative about which radiant source you connect with a particular system. For example, if I am juicing my spleen and pancreas to help support balanced blood sugar, I often plug into the heart of mother earth because it reminds my organs of all the energies available from foods and helps remind me sugar is not the only source of consolation. If I am juicing my third chakra (related to identity), I might plug into the radiance of a particular form of the Goddess.

You can combine this energy with "Bringing In Your Spirit Feeds" (page 156), plugging into your spirit-feed glyph, and using the "Divine Hook-Up" to steer that energy to a particular part of your body or mind.

• • • • • •

• • • EXERCISE: DUMBO • • •

Dumbo, the flying elephant, is a lovely symbol of our desire to lift out of the weighty, laden earth existence and find our wings to fly. Furthermore, elephants, with their long memory, symbolize our ability to remember all of who we have been in choosing who we wish to be moving forward.

Place your fingertips in a semicircular formation following the curve on the back of each ear. This area links your gatekeeper with its radiant nature. The triangles formed by each arm become your elephant ears and also your elephant *wings*. Slowly and luxuriantly flap those wing-ears, remembering to breathe. Imagine you are lifting into flight and traveling effortlessly through the air. Continue until you feel the desire to unfurl your elephant trunk and trumpet your joy to the heavens.

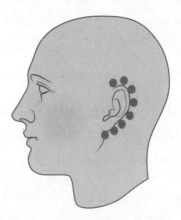

FIGURE 26. Place the fingertips behind the curve of the ear.

• • • • • •

• • • EXERCISE: HARMONIZING HOOK-UP • • •

This exercise involves using your hands to connect with your energetic grid; it allows deep radiance to enter, balance, and harmonize whatever energies need help. It can help reinforce your deepest energy systems, help knit together fragments of self, and generally fluff up your energies to move with greater ease and harmony. My inner teachers also claim that this exercise can help to connect you with a "universal energy grid" that transcends whatever disturbed patterns are moving through the earth energies at this time. It can bring you inner stability and a sense of security.

You can do it for yourself, but it is perhaps even more powerful if you try it with someone who cares about you and wishes you well.

Doing the Exercise with a Partner

Have the receiver lie faceup, in a comfortable position, where you can easily reach their left side. Place one hand flat on the front of their *left shoulder*, and the other hand flat on the front of their *left pelvis* (by the hip).

If you are the giving partner, open your feet to the earth, and open your head to the sky, and ask your partner to *hold hands with the Divine* (however that works for them). Then allow the energies to move through you, in silence, for at least three minutes. You do not have to control the energies or manage them or envision anything. I usually just watch and listen.

Often what happens is that the Divine energies come in and reinforce the deepest weave, shifting the polarities of the flow if needed. Sometimes it feels as if the person's aura gets fluffier and fuller, and their energy systems all begin to harmonize with one another. Often the person's sense of purpose and perspective will strengthen as well, as deep strands in their energy systems come together into a more harmonized whole.

For follow-up, I invite the client to hold hands with the Divine for five minutes a day for the next month, which allows the process to keep moving and integrating.

Doing the Exercise by Yourself

Lie down in a comfortable place, free from interruptions and distractions. Place one hand on the front of your left shoulder, the other hand on the front of your left pelvis by the hip, and since you have no hands free to hold hands with the Divine, imagine instead you are being rocked in the arms of the Divine, or you are gently swinging in a heavenly rainbow hammock.

Allow the energies to move and do what they will do for at least three to five minutes, and as with the partner version, follow up by holding hands with the Divine for five minutes a day (or at night) for up to a month.

• • • • • •

Other Exercises That Cultivate Radiance

All the meditations in this book help cultivate radiance, along with anything in everyday life that brings you home to your spirit.

Bringing In Your Spirit Feeds (page 156)
Exploring the Web of Meaning (page 31)
Cabinets of Wonders (page 79)
Core Note (page 96)
Core Shape (page 109)
Cosmic Figure Eight (page 158)
Clear Fear, Ease Ego, Welcome Wiser Self (page 148)
Divine Hook-Up (page 139)
Earth Dock–Sky Dock (page 212)
Twelve Hearts (page 222)
Seven Spirals (page 225)
Yin Hearts (page 198)
Five-Element Bed or Chair (page 176)

PRACTICE TIPS

Each of the six conversations discussed in chapters 10 and 11 offer a window into a whole slew of explorations. You can spend a month just focusing on one of the topics, or choose an exercise from each of the conversations to engage in daily.

You may want to use the following "Daily Energy Routine," which allows you to check in with the six conversations and gain insight, create better balance, and address at least briefly what needs to be invoked or supplied for greater well-being. Every day, try doing at least one exercise from each conversation.

Once you are familiar with the exercises, doing this daily energy routine can take as few as five minutes in order to rebalance your energies. You may want to use them in the morning to start your day in a balanced and conscious state. Or you might choose instead to use them throughout the day to support transitions or to bring you back home to yourself after work or before bed.

The exercises do not have to be done all at once — you can scatter them throughout your day as little energy breaks. The order can make a difference if you are feeling discombobulated: Calming the gatekeeper, grounding, and connecting your energies up all help you bring your instrument to a more optimal state. Then rebalancing your exchanges with the world, resetting your flows, and stepping into radiance help you to reset your ability to act in a more integrated and clear way.

On the other hand, you might have an instinct that you need a particular exercise at a specific juncture or feel guided to do them in a different order. In that case, follow your instinct!

The "Daily Energy Routine" includes a brief recap of how to do each exercise (as well as the page number where you can find the full version), so you can copy it and use it as a practice guide.

A DAILY ENERGY ROUTINE TO SUPPORT ENERGY DIALOGUE

To Support Your Gatekeeper

Do "Porcupine Reset" and "Inner Porcupine Reset" (page 201), "Yin Hearts" (page 198), and "Reinforcing the Smart Filter of the Aura" (page 205).

Porcupine Reset

1. Grasp the "sky energy" at the top of your head. With an inhale, pull both arms straight up.
2. With an exhale, arc each arm outward, pulling the energy downward and tacking it to the floor.
3. With an inhale, grab "earth energy" and pull it in an outward arc up toward the top of your head.
4. With an exhale, tack the earth energy to the top of your head.

Inner Porcupine Reset

Repeat the same pattern as "Porcupine Reset," but begin and end at the third eye.

Yin Hearts

Slowly and lovingly trace at least three hearts over the area of your anatomical heart.

Reinforcing the Smart Filter of the Aura

1. Figure-eight toward and away from you with arms extended, sending your intentions to the edge of your aura.
2. Reinforce your smart filter with a color and invite helpers to figure-eight the entire egg-shaped edge of your aura all the way around, above, and below you.

To Ground, Root, and Anchor

Do "Earth Dock–Sky Dock" (page 212).

Earth Dock–Sky Dock

1. Stand with legs apart and inhale. On the exhale, send taproots down from the K-1 points on the bottoms of your feet, eight feet below the earth's surface to dock on the stabilized shelf.

2. Inhale again and draw stabilized energy up through your body (using your hands to help it move), and while exhaling, send it up through the top of your head and into the heavens to dock on the star with your name on it.

3. Inhale and use your hands to guide your star energy down into your body, exhaling and using your hands to send it down to meet your earth-docked roots.

4. Now use either hand to figure-eight the five-pointed star:

   • Between your earth-docked right foot and the sky dock (water-fire)

   • Between your sky dock and earth-docked left foot (fire-metal)

   • Between your left-foot dock and extended right hand (metal-wood)

   • Between your right hand and extended left hand (wood-earth)

   • Between your extended left hand and your right-foot dock (earth-water)

5. Now trace your whole earth-docked, sky-docked being with clockwise circles (right side to head to left side to feet). Repeat several circles to promote flow.

To Promote Inner Connection and Coherence

Do either "Twelve Hearts" (page 222) or "Sing a Scale" (page 222).

Twelve Hearts

1. Slowly and with radiance, place your hands on your heart chakra.

2. Then trace 3 hearts around the face and anchor each at the heart.

3. Trace 3 hearts around the upper torso area and anchor each at the heart chakra.

4. Trace 3 hearts around the pelvic bowl and anchor each at the belly button.

5. Return hands to the heart chakra, then trace three hearts that encompass your entire energy field.

Sing a Scale

1. If you know your core note, begin and end with that note. Otherwise, start with any note you wish.

2. Sing a full octave up, then back down again.

To Create Right Relationship with the World

Do "Seven Spirals" (page 225).

Seven Spirals

With either palm (or both) facing the named direction, circle first one way, then the other in the following directions: in front of you, behind you, above you, below you, to the left, to the right, and within (toward your heart).

To Reset Your Energy Flows

Do "Suit Reboot" (page 230).

Suit Reboot

1. Imagine your body is a large snowsuit. Unzip it, pull off the sleeves, and step out of the suit.

2. Turn around and pick up the suit by the feet. Shake it gently to remove any wrinkles.

3. Dip your suit in the "Well of Resolution" to dissolve all unwanted energies and reset the circuits.

4. Place your suit upright behind you and step back into it, one

leg at a time, then place each arm in its sleeve, pull the hood over your head, and zip it up.

To Bring In Radiance

Do one of the following three exercises: "Dumbo" (page 234), "Clear Fear, Ease Ego, Welcome Wiser Self" (page 148), or "Harmonizing Hook-Up" (page 235).

Dumbo

1. Cup the fingertips of each hand around the curve behind each ear, creating elephant ears.
2. Then slowly and majestically flap your wing-ears until you feel yourself achieve liftoff.

Clear Fear, Ease Ego, Welcome Wiser Self

1. Do a "Divine Hook-Up," plugging one index finger into your "gamut point" on the back of your hand (between the fourth and fifth fingers below the knuckles) and the other index finger into the "heart of the Divine." Hold for at least five breaths.
2. Then plug one index finger into your heart, and the other into the heart of the Divine and hold.
3. Finally, massage your Ming-men area (at the L4-L5 vertebrae); flip your hand back and forth a few times over the Ming-men. Then invite your Wiser Self to connect with you there and to step forward to meld with you (or you can step back to meld with it).

Harmonizing Hook-Up

1. Place one hand flat on the front of your left shoulder; the other palm flat on your left pelvis beside the hip.
2. Imagine yourself held in the arms of the Divine, and hold that connection for at least three minutes, allowing the Divine radiance to permeate every level of your being.

CONCLUSION

Coming Full Circle

Energy dialogue is an ongoing practice of engaging with your subtle energies in partnership and friendship. It does not ask that you have a huge vocabulary or toolbox full of tools (though a good number are on offer in this book). It does ask that you meet your own creation of self with an open mind and heart and a willingness to listen, learn, and respond with sensitive support.

The rewards when you do this are often immediate and sometimes miraculous. Even when there is no response, or the conversation requires a back-and-forth over time, you will get a sense of rightness, of being on your path. Just showing up is potent medicine. Turning off the socialized mind to listen to the authentic voices within will activate your own inner healer. Using your outsider perspective to see yourself as a web of meaning rather than a chemistry project will allow you to participate more fully in your larger, glorious creation of self!

If you find yourself saying: "Yes, yes, I get all that, and I read this whole book, but I am feeling *sick*. My symptoms block me from participating in anything large or glorious. Where do I start, what do I do?" The answer is: Start with your breath. Follow that for a time and support the rhythms of it. Then let your healing hands go where they want to go to initiate a conversation in the language of touch (see "Healing Hands," page 74). Take logic out of the equation for a time and let your creative, intuitive self guide your motions and energy dialogue.

Healing is not linear, and sometimes when we get too focused on the problem — trying to find out *why* we have the symptoms, or what the illness means in the larger picture — we miss the communication of a body asking us to meet it moment by moment. When your mind is trying too hard to steer the ship or attack the problem, let your heart and Wiser Self and body wisdom guide you to a different place, where you can see things from a different perspective. Taking care of just *one* need in a moment — for water, for rest, for respite, for retreat, for taking a small risk, for exhale or release, for consolation, for acceptance — will get the ship moving so it can be steered from within. Trying to steer while standing still is almost impossible!

You can use this book as a kind of divination tool. Ask your Wiser Self to guide you to what is needed *now*. Then open the book at random and read the text or suggestions. Pick one of the "Play With It" sections to just pull you into an activity of exploration and dialogue.

Befriend your gatekeeper. If you are in a stuck or panicked place, first do something to calm the gatekeeper ("Porcupine Reset," page 201; "Yin Hearts," page 198; "Clear Fear, Ease Ego, Welcome Wiser Self," page 148). Then, when your gatekeeper is a bit calmer, ask yourself what gifts the symptoms and illness bring, what screwy purpose they serve. Address your gatekeeper's four concerns: safety, identity, distribution of resources, and managing the autopilot templates. Call on your gatekeeper's cosmic partner, radiance, to help shift the conversation.

Remember that illness is usually not just a signal that something is wrong. It also signals that something *right* is missing. Instead of asking, "What is wrong and how can I fix it?" learn to ask: "What is needed and how can I lovingly supply it?" Bringing in what is right activates an urge on the part of your body, mind, and spirit to seek even more rightness. If you need release first, to make space for new energy to come in, develop gestures that accomplish that. Then invoke what is needed in this moment.

Ongoing dialogue builds trust, relationship, and communion over time. In terms of your subtle energies, ongoing energy dialogue builds resilience and a stronger core, better circulation and coherence, and more effective grounding. Over a period of time, try the "Daily Energy Routine" (page 238). With each exercise, tune in to see what you can perceive about your subtle energies, do the exercise, and then do it again, invoking whatever quality your inner self is craving.

True communication is an ongoing conversation, not a single morning or evening routine. Enhance your day with energy snacks, moments of attention and support for transitions, and recognition of when your energy flows are faltering and need attention.

Play with your energies, speak their language, dance with them, and they will teach you how to find your way home to your fully realized, vibrant self.

EXERCISES AND MEDITATIONS

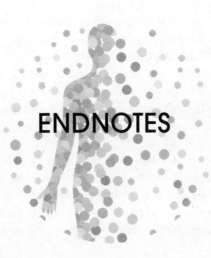

ENDNOTES

1. Donna Eden and David Feinstein, *Energy Medicine: Balancing Your Body's Energies for Optimal Health, Joy, and Vitality* (New York: Jeremy P. Tarcher/Penguin, 2008), 4.

2. For more about Ruth Denison, visit www.ruthdenison.com. Also see Sandy Boucher, *Dancing in the Dharma: The Life and Teachings of Ruth Denison* (Boston: Beacon Press, 2008).

3. Donna Eden and David Feinstein, *Advanced Chakra Work* (Ashland, OR: Inner-source, 2015), DVD.

4. For more information on Touch for Health, visit the website (http://touchforhealth .us) or read John Thie and Matthew Thie, *Touch for Health: A Practical Guide to Natural Health with Acupressure Touch* (Camarillo, CA: DeVorss & Co, 2005).

5. These are adapted loosely from Donna Eden and David Feinstein, "Principles of Energy Medicine," Energy Medicine Handout Bank, 2012, http://energymed.org /hbank/handouts/principles_ener_med.htm.

6. This is explored more extensively in my book: Ellen Meredith, *Listening In: Dialogues with the Wiser Self* (Haydenville, MA: Horse Mountain Press, 1993).

7. These techniques are part of the "Cosmic Reset" in my four-DVD set: Ellen Meredith, *Gatekeeper: Energy Medicine for the Immune System and Energetic Reactivity* (Haydenville, MA: Horse Mountain Press, 2012), DVD, available at www.listening-in .com/gatekeeper.php.

8. For more on template clearing, see my four-DVD set: Ellen Meredith, *Storyline*

Track and Balance: Clearing Energy Habits Where They Live (Haydenville, MA: Horse Mountain Press, 2012), DVD, available at www.listening-in.com/storyline.php.

9.   Bruce Lipton, *The Biology of Belief, Unleashing the Power of Consciousness, Matter, and Miracles* (Carlsbad, CA: Hay House, 2015).

10.   Gratitude to Sarah J. Buck, who first woke me up to the possibility of drawing the five-pointed star on the body to communicate with the five elements within us.

11.   Thanks to Sandra Huisinga for her creative insights in using the star this way.

12.   For an excellent introduction to a syntax of nine major energy systems, see Eden and Feinstein, *Energy Medicine.*

13.   At that time I used Donna Eden's daily energy routine, which is an excellent starting place and baseline practice. See Donna Eden, "Donna Eden's Daily Energy Routine," YouTube, posted November 24, 2015, https://www.youtube.com/watch?v=Di5Ua44iuXc. Over time I created the daily energy routine presented in this chapter.

14.   For more information on this topic, see Body Ecology by Donna Gates, https://body ecology.com.

15.   Gratitude to Paulette Taschereau, EEMAP, for contributing this part of the protocol!

16.   Thank you to Stephanie Eldringhoff for teaching this exercise.

17.   For more on this topic, see Traditional Chinese Medicine World Foundation, "Meridian Connection," https://www.tcmworld.org/what-is-tcm/meridian-connection; and Cathy Wong, "Meridians in Acupuncture and Chinese Medicine," Very Well Health, September 1, 2019, https://www.verywellhealth.com/what-are-meridians -88946.

18.   To learn how to trace your meridians and tune in to them specifically, see Donna Eden, "Tracing Meridians with Donna Eden!," YouTube, posted September 28, 2017, https://www.youtube.com/watch?v=Vv5dkvMg1z4. Or search online for "tracing meridians."

19.   See note 13 above.

ACKNOWLEDGMENTS

I want to acknowledge you, the reader, with gratitude for being willing to explore energy dialogue and deepen your ability to heal. This book is meant to be a companion for you as you relearn how to communicate with your body-mind-spirit in the language of energy. May the tools and frameworks in this book serve you well. I truly believe that each time you make an effort to reclaim your first language, energy, you are enriching the web of connection that feeds all beings.

Many people were instrumental and sometimes unwittingly incidental in helping me find this work and give it shape. Judith L. Evans, my life partner, helped me keep body, mind, and soul together when they wanted to go in different directions. She has grounded me and supported me for forty-two years and counting. Donna Eden has been my teacher, mentor, friend, and sistah and my inspiration in codifying my own understandings of the language of energy. If I quote her too many times in this book, it is because I believe her work is so foundational and important! Paulette Taschereau has been my faithful foil, coteacher, friend, and sounding board through the ups and downs of bringing this perspective on energy healing into form.

This book is better because of the comments and support (and some criticism) from my early readers: Judith Evans, Patricia Yeghissian, Gabriel Gilbert, Jean Ball, Paulette Taschereau, Amy Schill, Donna Eden, David Feinstein, Devi Stern, and Jaime Schwalb. Thank you!

I thank my mom for giving me an ear for language, and my dad for his tin ear that forced me to trust my own hearing, and my dead grandmother who while alive was sweet and loving, and who, once dead, woke me up to things I hadn't considered. I also thank my Councils for their ongoing guidance.

Steve Harris, my awesome agent, made the process of finding the right home for this book painless and quick. I am so grateful to have found New World Library through his agency.

I am deeply grateful to my visionary editor, Georgia Hughes, for believing in this book and helping me get it to its best self. I also want to thank Jeff Campbell, copyeditor, for his valiant efforts to tame my erratic usage and his insights on format that made this book clearer. I am grateful to Kristen Cashman for her editorial oversight, and to Kim Corbin for wise guidance on how to spread the word. Everyone at New World Library is awesome. I feel blessed to have landed this book in their capable hands.

The material and perspectives in this book were brewed over years of interactions and experiences with healers, clients, students, friends, colleagues, and even chance encounters with strangers. I thank all of you for teaching me. I also want to thank in particular: Barbara Allen; Francey and Laurel Liefert; Richard Lalli; Sandy Wand; Nancy Manyi-Ten Williamson; Melinda Jacobs; the faculty of the Eden Energy Medicine Certification Program, especially Barb Scholz, Jeff Harris, Adriana Barraza, Debra Burchard, Janie Chandler, Doug Moore, Donna Kemper, Sara Allen, Susan Stone, Melanie Smith, and Margie Fein; my WWWW support group; and class organizers: Sarah J. Buck, Emily Butler, Donna Racik, Ann Deatly, June Scott, Julie Fowler, Susan Stone, and the Ft. Myers trio. Also, Diane and Stuart Friebert, Güneli Gun, Sandy Boucher, Ruth Denison, Kathy Lewis, and the Chetwood gals. There are more, but the house orchestra is playing loud music to get me off the stage!

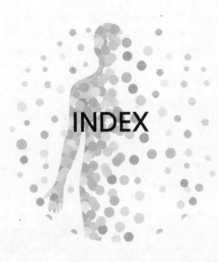

INDEX

When multiple references for exercises are given, page references in **bold** indicate instructions for how to perform the exercise.

ABOUT THE AUTHOR

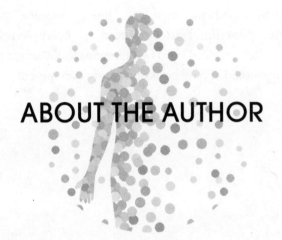

Ellen Meredith, Doctor of Arts, is a conscious channel, medical intuitive, energy medicine practitioner, teacher, writer, traveler, framer, storyteller, and visionary. She has been in practice since 1984, helping over ten thousand clients and students across the globe tune in to and communicate with their own energies, hear their inner guidance, and heal.

Ellen is renowned for her down-to-earth yet out-of-the-box thinking. Her approach to self-healing with energy medicine offers readers ways to understand and get to the heart of their health and life challenges and to work compassionately with their body, mind, and spiritual dimensions. She builds on everyday experiences and commonsense frameworks, believing that life reveals more of its meaning if you treat it as an evolving story and see yourself as a unique character helping to cocreate it.

Originally trained as a healer by her inner teachers (Councils), Ellen later became an Eden Energy Medicine Advanced Practitioner (EEMAP) and served on Donna Eden's faculty. She brings humanity, humor, and insight in many forms to the world of energy healing. Ellen is the author of *Listening In: Dialogues with the Wiser Self,* the audiobook *In Search of Radiance: Learning to Stand with Your Wiser Self*, and numerous video classes on energy medicine, including "Energy Fluency," "Gatekeeper," "Energy Chiro," "Storyline Track and Balance," "Energy Wisdom," "Intuition and Practioner's Mind" and "Healing Spaces." Using a pseudonym, she has also published several books on child development.

www.ellenmeredith.com